Selling the Fountain of Youth

Selling the Fountain of Youth

How the Anti-Aging
Industry Made a
Disease out of
Getting Old—
and Made Billions

ARLENE WEINTRAUB

BASIC
BOOKS
A MEMBER OF THE PERSEUS BOOKS GROUP
New York

Books published by Basic Books are available at special discounts
for bulk purchases in the United States by corporations,
institutions, and other organizations. For more information, please
contact the Special Markets Department at the Perseus Books
Group, 2300 Chestnut Street, Suite 200, Philadelphia, PA 19103, or
call (800) 810-4145, ext. 5000, or e-mail
special.markets@perseusbooks.com.

Library of Congress Cataloging-in-Publication Data
Weintraub, Arlene.
    Selling the fountain of youth : how the anti-aging industry made
a disease out of getting old—and made billions / Arlene
Weintraub.
        p. ; cm.
    Includes index.
    ISBN 978–0-465–01721–8
    1. Longevity. 2. Pharmaceutical industry. 3. Somatotropin. 4.
Hormones, Sex. I. Title.
[DNLM: 1. Aging—United States. 2. Drug Therapy—history—
United States. 3. Drug Industry—economics—United States. 4.
Drug Industry—history—United States. 5. History, 20th
Century—United States. 6. History, 21st Century—United States. 7.
Rejuvenation—United States. WT 11 AA1 W424s 2010]
    RA776.75.W45 2010
    338.4'76151—dc22

                                                2010003369

10 9 8 7 6 5 4 3 2 1

CONTENTS

I will follow that system of regimen which, according to my ability and judgment, I consider for the benefit of my patients, and abstain from whatever is deleterious and mischievous.

—HIPPOCRATIC OATH

When we replace the missing hormones in older people—replace them to the level of younger people—a very exciting thing happens. Cells start to respond and actually grow younger in terms of their physiology and in terms of their function.

—DR. RONALD KLATZ, PRESIDENT, THE
AMERICAN ACADEMY OF ANTI-AGING
MEDICINE, AS QUOTED ON
WWW.THIRDAGE.COM

PREFACE

I first wandered into the odd world of anti-aging medicine while working as a science writer for *BusinessWeek*. It was 2005, and I was reporting a story on a new wave of drugs designed to help children who couldn't grow properly. The biotechnology innovation known as human growth hormone (HGH) was the most widely accepted treatment for these children, and parents were still clamoring for it. But as I called various doctors to report the story, some of them told me they were disturbed about an entirely different trend they were seeing: Aging adults wanted to take HGH, too.

I wondered, why would any fully grown adult need growth hormone? That single question opened my eyes to an emerging specialty called anti-aging medicine. The deeper I dug, the more fascinated I became with the bizarre and ever-growing medicine chest of drugs anti-aging doctors were prescribing— and the hordes of patients who seemed to have no idea that these treatments could be seriously risky.

In 2006, I wrote a cover story for *BusinessWeek* called "Forever Young: Selling the Promise of Youth," which questioned the claims anti-aging doctors were making about HGH and other substances they prescribed. That story attracted many more reader responses than anything else I have ever written.

Some patients who had tried anti-aging regimens e-mailed me with horror stories about side effects they had suffered. Others defended their anti-aging habits. One man even called me to beg for the phone number of the anti-aging doctor who was the main character in my piece. (I refused.)

I knew I had much more to say about anti-aging medicine. Most of all, I wanted to set out my views about what seemed to be outrageous promises anti-aging doctors were making.

To research this book, I spent several months interviewing and shadowing the best-known doctors in the field of anti-aging medicine, as well as some of their patients. I spent time with the entrepreneurs who started chains of anti-aging clinics, and I attended conferences put on by the American Academy of Anti-Aging Medicine and its rival, Age Management Medicine Group. I scoured literature on hormone replacement and interviewed scientists and doctors who were trying—mostly in vain—to warn patients away from the most heavily touted regimens.

None of my reporting was done under cover; every person I interviewed knew that I was a journalist. Although I did submit myself to an anti-aging workup while reporting the *BusinessWeek* story, I never tried any of the drugs or supplements that were recommended to me. By the time you get to the end of the book, you should understand why.

Anti-aging doctors believe they're acting in good faith and truly helping patients. I understand that. Yet most of what these physicians present to patients are rosy promises about hormone replacement—promises that are not always well supported by scientific evidence. This book is my chance to present the other side of the story. I have examined the facts and laid out my conclusions in these pages.

All quotations in this book were said to me or to my research assistant, unless otherwise noted. All quotations from books are accurate according to the editions I consulted. Most importantly, all patients and relatives of patients who appear here are real. I urge anyone who is tempted to try anti-aging remedies to read their stories and learn from them.

And remember this: Sometimes doctors are wrong.

CHAPTER 1

"Physician, Heal Thyself!"

You wake up on Monday, bound out of bed, head for the medicine cabinet, and grab a syringe filled with human growth hormone. With no hesitation, you stick the needle into a fold of skin on your thigh and press the plunger. Then you open a tube of estrogen cream that you bought from the neighborhood pharmacist and rub a dollop of it into your arm. You're 56 years old, but your hot flashes are a distant nightmare, and you wake up with the energy of a 20-year-old. You attribute your newfound youth not only to the growth hormone and the estrogen but also to the sleep-promoting hormone melatonin, which you take every night. You've heard that some hormones can cause cancer, but you're not too worried. Your doctor at the local anti-aging clinic told you the cancer fears are overblown. You're just replacing the hormones your body made naturally when you were younger, he says. There's nothing dangerous about that, right? If there were, surely all the 20-year-olds would have cancer!

Before you leave for work, you head for the kitchen, where you whip up a fruit smoothie and gulp it down with 35 supplement pills. You take a multivitamin that was made just for you by the pharmacist, plus dozens of herbal preparations that he told you would guarantee a long life. You're getting your menstrual period again, because your anti-aging doctor told you to cycle your estrogen with progesterone—changing the dosage week by week to mimic what your body did when you were in your prime. It would do so much more than relieve your hot flashes, he promised. It would make you feel young again. The famous actress Suzanne Somers takes hormones like this, too, and she says she feels fantastic. She would never give out dumb advice, right?

The pharmacist said his hormone creams were completely natural, made from vegetables, and so much safer than those dangerous menopause drugs the pharmaceutical companies make. Neither his products nor his advertising claims are monitored by government agencies, but why should you care? He's a pharmacist—he would never sell anything unhealthy, right? And at least he doesn't expect you to pore over any pesky product leaflets about side effects.

During your last checkup at the anti-aging clinic, you found out that your lab tests show abnormally high levels of the male hormone testosterone. Your doctor said it rubbed off on you when you were intimate with your husband—something you've been in the mood for a lot more often since you started your hormone treatments. Your husband was very impressed with the new you, so he made an appointment at the anti-aging clinic, too. He told them that he felt a little tired and that his libido was sagging. They prescribed some testosterone gel to restore his virility. And boy, did that testosterone work wonders for your sex life.

As you pour your husband a smoothie, you wonder if it matters that his testosterone gel is rubbing off on you. Sure, most women don't have so much testosterone, and you did notice some hair growing in weird places. But lots of women use testosterone gel these days to restore the libidinous urges they had in their youth. Plus, it's a natural hormone, just like what's found in our bodies normally. It's perfectly safe. Right?

Welcome to the new world of anti-aging medicine. It emerged in the 1990s and is promoted with a deceptively simple but incredibly appealing sales pitch: Hormones rage when we're young and then wane as we age. Therefore we can stop the aging process by replacing the hormones we've lost over the years. In essence, we can reset our bodies to their younger selves. The rapidly expanding group of doctors, pharmacists, and entrepreneurs who promote this brand of medicine do much more than erase wrinkles and make varicose veins disappear. Instead, they focus on using drugs to try to stop the biological clock from deep inside the human body. Hormones are the primary building blocks of this new fountain of youth.

Anti-aging medicine may be misguided. And it could be dangerous. But it has grown into an $88-billion-a-year industry in little more than a decade. A small portion of that growth comes from cosmetic products to make us look more youthful, such as the antiwrinkle drug Botox and laser-based skin treatments. But the vast majority of these receipts emanate from high-priced doctors and rogue pharmacists selling expensive, unproven drugs. Some practitioners have promised women that they can bypass menopause by taking estrogens that are more natural than what pharmaceutical companies offer.

Others have assured men that they can safely regain the sexual prowess they enjoyed in their twenties by taking a little testosterone and growth hormone every day. Still others have transformed Chinese herbs and Brazilian berries into miraculous youth-restoring elixirs—and suckered millions of patients into buying expensive subscriptions to have those concoctions delivered right to their doorsteps.

All this marketing muscle, of course, is aimed at treating a nonexistent malady. Getting old is not a disease. The U.S. Food and Drug Administration (FDA) has never approved any therapy to treat aging. And although mainstream medical organizations have issued plenty of guidelines for preventing illnesses that commonly occur late in life, such as heart disease and cancer, none has ever fully endorsed the treatment regimens that the anti-aging industry embraces.

Nevertheless, anti-aging doctors have persuaded millions of baby boomers that they can stop the inevitable march toward Metamucil mornings and Viagra nights. These capitalists have constructed a giant new industry by taking advantage of an entire generation's deep-seated aversion to getting old. Their task has been made that much easier by the American culture, which has slapped images of beautiful young people all over movie and television screens, newspapers, and magazines. For the nation's 77 million baby boomers, who are quickly racing toward the Social Security rolls, the idea of being elderly is repugnant. They are the perfect audience for the message that simple, safe substances might cure aging.

Every generation in history has embarked on its own search for the fountain of youth. Legends about magical potions with age-defying powers date back to ancient Greece. Spanish explorer Juan Ponce de León popularized the quest for longevity in the 1500s, when he surmised that a spring on an island near what is now Florida would restore youth to anyone who sipped its waters.

What makes the modern anti-aging movement different is the loud enthusiasm with which it is promoted. Most of the doctors who have hung out shingles in anti-aging medicine did so after dabbling in hormones themselves and being so wowed by their own results that they passed on their new-found passion to other youth seekers.

Among the claims made by proponents of anti-aging products: Soybeans are a healthy source of estrogen because they make the hormone just like people do. Drugs mixed up in the back rooms of tiny pharmacies are safer than those manufactured in quality-controlled, government-supervised factories. Hormones are unnatural and dangerous when they are extracted from horses but perfectly harmless when they come from pigs. The list goes on. The seemingly twisted logic of these claims makes the anti-aging movement appear to be more a cult than a medical specialty.

The modern anti-aging movement actually started on the opposite end of the age spectrum, with children. Short children, to be exact. Growth hormone is produced by the body's "master gland," the pituitary, which works overtime in the first years of life to transform a child into an adult. Children with defective pituitary glands don't grow properly. Doctors once treated these youngsters with growth hormone harvested from cadavers, but supplies were scarce. Then, in the 1970s, scientists at the University of California at San Francisco and startup Genentech invented a gene-splicing technique that allowed them to produce growth hormone in bacteria. This feat of genetic engineering, which was called "recombinant DNA," became the basis of the multi-billion-dollar biotechnology industry. Human growth hormone (HGH) was among the first of the newfangled drugs that the fledgling industry produced on a massive scale.

Long before HGH became a marketable product, a handful of scientists around the country began thinking about the drug's potential to reach a much bigger market—aging baby boomers. Among them was Daniel Rudman, a scientist at Emory University who specialized in endocrinology, the study of hormones. The aging of the endocrine system, and the resulting loss of hormones, fascinated Rudman. He knew growth hormone was particularly vital for keeping adults healthy, even after they reached their normal height. It helped maintain a proper balance of fat mass and lean mass and of good to bad cholesterol. It preserved bone density and stimulated the immune system. Adults with severe growth hormone deficiencies suffered a range of problems, from increased fractures to debilitating fatigue. But Rudman thought HGH might be useful as more than just a treatment for those gravely sick individuals. HGH, he thought, might just be the new fountain of youth.

In 1980, regulators at the FDA realized that synthetic hormones would soon become a reality. So they gathered together a panel of experts, including Rudman, to advise the agency. According to a *New York Times* article, Rudman raved about the hormone's potential for building muscle and for restoring the tissues of the liver, kidney, and heart. Scientists around the world began designing studies to investigate the potential of HGH as a panacea against aging.

In 1985, the FDA approved Genentech's HGH to treat growth disorders in children. It would eventually green-light the drug for the treatment of severe growth hormone deficiencies in adults and in some AIDS patients. Pfizer, Eli Lilly, and a handful of other big pharma companies began selling HGH, too.

Federal legislators feared that HGH might be abused by athletes hoping to improve their muscle tone. So the government would eventually take the rare step of making it illegal for doctors to prescribe HGH "off-label"—that is, for any use the FDA had not sanctioned. Some anti-aging medicine seems to fall into that verboten category.

Despite the percolating controversy, Rudman was determined to test his hypothesis that HGH might reverse aging. So the scientist, who moved to the Medical College of Wisconsin in 1988, assembled a group of ten scientists to design a study. They placed newspaper ads soliciting healthy older men for the trial and interviewed everyone who volunteered. They ended up with a group of 21, ranging in age from 61 to 81. Twelve of the men were given injections of HGH. Over six months, those men increased their lean body mass, including muscle, by 9 percent, on average. They lost 14 percent of their fat. "Diminished secretion of growth hormone is responsible in part for the decrease of lean body mass, the expansion of adipose-tissue mass, and the thinning of the skin that occurs in old age," Rudman wrote in a paper summarizing the study, "Effects of Human Growth Hormone in Men over 60 Years Old." The problem could be solved, he posited, "by the administration of human growth hormone."

Rudman's study was printed in the July 5, 1990, edition of the prestigious *New England Journal of Medicine.* When the Internet became popular a few years later, Rudman's words were resurrected and spread around with abandon. The study was quoted on more than 50,000 Web sites, some belonging to Internet pharmacies that were selling HGH illegally.

Ronald Klatz was among the legions impressed by Rudman's research. Klatz was working at a medical clinic in Wisconsin as a doctor of osteopathic medicine—a type of internist. He was only in his mid-thirties, but when he looked in the mirror, he could see the aging process starting. "I said, physician, heal thyself!" Klatz recalled in a 2006 interview. Then, in 1992, Klatz suffered a cervical fracture in a car accident and was forced to go on disability leave, according to the *New York Times*. Backed by $500,000 in disability payments, he conceived of a new medical movement, based on the tenet that hormones could prevent the ravages of old age. He recalled in 2006, "Ninety percent of disease is chronic and degenerative, so that's where I decided to plant my target. What is the bull's-eye? Aging."

Klatz teamed up with an old friend and fellow osteopath, Robert Goldman. A fitness nut, Goldman often showed off photos of himself as a curly-haired youth, dressed in nothing but checkered briefs, setting world records of 321 consecutive handstand push-ups and 161 one-arm push-ups. He was active in the International Federation of Body Building and Fitness and often hobnobbed with famous musclemen, such as Arnold Schwarzenegger. More gregarious than Klatz, Goldman would become an influential proselytizer of anti-aging medicine.

The two doctors set up shop in a Gothic-looking building in Lincoln Park, a ritzy Chicago neighborhood filled with upscale boutiques and exclusive restaurants. The citizens of Lincoln Park were mostly white and had a median household income of about $80,000 a year—just the type of people who would be drawn to anti-aging medicine.

In 1993, Klatz and Goldman found a new ally in Howard Turney, a business executive who was so intrigued by Rudman's paper that he started traveling back and forth to Mexico to buy vials of HGH for himself. "At 59, I was all used up," Turney recalled years later. He was exhausted, he said, and disgusted by the belly fat forming in his midsection. His right hand shook uncontrollably. "I looked like my father. I had a god-awful amount of loose skin. In general, I was a mess." Five months into his HGH treatments, Turney said, his hand stopped shaking, his fat started to disappear, and his muscles were growing. And he hadn't changed a thing about his exercise habits or diet. "I had worn bifocals for 20 years," he said. "One day I picked up the *Wall Street Journal* and I was reading the stock report without them."

Turney was determined to share his HGH discovery, so he quit his job and opened the El Dorado Clinic in Playa del Carmen, Mexico, in February 1993. El Dorado, named for the fabled city of gold, offered HGH as the shiny path to a long and prosperous life. The clinic's doctors taught guests how to inject themselves with HGH. "Our deal was, people paid $4,600 for the exam, a three-month supply of HGH, and three nights in the hotel," Turney said. He started placing ads in publications such as *Robb Report*, the magazine for millionaires.

Turney heard that Klatz and Goldman were launching a new medical society to promote HGH, so he invited them to El Dorado's grand opening in November 1993. Klatz and Goldman turned the occasion into the first scientific meeting of their brand-new organization, the American Academy of Anti-Aging Medicine (A4M). There, in a mansion on the beach— surrounded by smiling 50-somethings who were learning how to inject themselves with HGH—a small group of doctors established a mission for A4M. They would certify doctors in their new specialty, they decided, and hold conferences to discuss the latest science of anti-aging medicine. "They took that thing and built it into quite an organization," Turney said.

Klatz described the El Dorado meeting in his 1997 book *Grow Young with HGH*. "Anti-aging medicine—the slowing down, stopping, or even reversing the downward course of senescence—seemed to us an idea whose time had truly come," Klatz wrote. He marveled at the "sexy, energetic, upbeat" people who were guests at the spa. "They talked about changes they had undergone—melting away of fat, increased muscle tone even in the absence of exercise, rapid healing from surgery, disappearance of wrinkles and cellulite, a vastly increased sense of well-being." It was all because of HGH, he claimed. Klatz dedicated the book to Rudman, who had died in 1994, and hailed the HGH research as "remarkably prescient." As for the 12 men who got HGH during the study, Klatz declared, they were pioneers. "The invincibility of the aging process had been shattered once and for all," Klatz wrote. "Like the first people to have received cow pox vaccine, or the first heart transplant recipients, these twelve men had changed the course of history forever."

Rudman's experiment fell far short of what some scientists would consider compelling justification for using HGH to halt aging. True scientific proof, equivalent to what the FDA demands before it will approve drugs for specific diseases, requires years of testing on thousands of patients. Some of those patients should be given a placebo or some other treatment, and none should be told whether they're getting the real drug or a fake. The doctors recording the reactions of study subjects shouldn't know who's getting the real drug, either. Such studies are known in scientific circles as "randomized," "double-blind," and "placebo-controlled," and they are the gold standard of evidence gathering. But Rudman's study wasn't even close: His control group got nothing, and the entire cohort was way too small to draw any meaningful conclusions about HGH in healthy aging people.

The many doctors who followed Klatz into anti-aging medicine accepted this imperfect research. They didn't have much choice: Few studies of hormones were randomized, controlled, or lengthy enough to draw conclusions about their safety and usefulness as anti-aging tools. That's because it would be challenging to recruit patients to participate in such research. What sane person, after all, would volunteer for a study where he or she might end up taking a placebo for years on end rather than the hormone that might extend life? And who would agree to be exposed to hormones for years when so little was known about how safe it was to do so? The lack of rigorous research presented a conundrum: For every trial such as Rudman's that suggested hormone use was safe for healthy people, there were other studies that indicated just the opposite. The anti-aging industry had a knack for finding—and heavily promoting—the evidence that appeared to validate their therapies.

Klatz was fond of telling stories about real people who said HGH changed their lives. In his book, he wrote about El Dorado's founder, Turney, and about Paul Bernstein, a 64-year-old who enjoyed injecting HGH, as did his 53-year-old wife. "The awesome power of GH to bring about total rejuvenation unlike any medicine that has ever existed can perhaps be appreciated by the stories of the people who have experienced it firsthand," Klatz asserted.

Klatz devoted an entire chapter to Edmund Chein, a California doctor who, at age 42, decided to give himself the hormone profile of a 20-year-old. He started taking HGH and four other hormones, and claimed to have cured his cholesterol and weight problems within six months. Turney's clinic inspired Chein to start up an HGH center in the United States. Klatz wrote, "doctors now routinely prescribe aspirin to thin the blood and prevent heart attacks. Yet its approved use is as an anti-inflammatory drug for headaches, pain, and fever." He described Chein's thought process: "It is much further afield, he points out, to use aspirin for heart disease than to use growth hormone for aging."

To test his HGH treatment plan, Chein teamed up with a former Rudman colleague, L. Cass Terry, a neurologist who was also taking HGH. Together they analyzed symptoms and blood tests from 800 patients who visited Chein's clinic between 1994 and 1996, Klatz said in his book. The research had not been published in a peer-reviewed journal, which would have required scrutiny and sign-offs from independent scientists. Nevertheless, Klatz printed the study, complete with charts and tables. But there was no control group, so everyone in the study was taking HGH. And the reported responses to the drug were mostly the self-described observations of 202 of the patients. The results were stunning: Patients reported an 88 percent improvement in muscle strength, an 84 percent boost in energy, and a 75 percent improvement in sexual prowess.

Klatz seemed to downplay the side effects. Some patients in Chein and Terry's study suffered minor pains and fluid retention, but those annoyances went away after a couple of months, Klatz wrote. And even though some scientists worried that growth hormone might cause cancer to grow, Klatz said, there were no reported cases of cancer among the 800 patients. Surmised Terry, "It could be that there is some sort of protective effect from growth hormone replacement."

By the late 1990s, Klatz and Goldman were luring 3,000 visitors a day to A4M's Web site, which they dubbed the World Health Network. They launched their own publication and called it the *International Journal of Anti-Aging Medicine.* On their Web site, they posted a "longevity test"—a multiple-choice quiz that purported to tell people how long they would live. Klatz and Goldman did not understate their goals for the new medical society: "Anti-aging medicine will be the most profound social and economic issue of the 21st century," they wrote, "restructuring and redirecting the trillion dollar plus a year economics of health care in radical new ways."

Klatz and Goldman appeared to be on the leading edge of a hot trend. By the mid-1990s, the first of the baby boomers were turning 50. And the consumer-products industry eagerly embraced the term "anti-aging" as a way to sell products to help them hide their age. In 1994, Revlon launched its Age Defying makeup collection. That same year, Avon introduced Anew, a line of cosmetics with names like Rejuvenate and Advanced Wrinkle Corrector. Anti-aging was a catchphrase with selling power: Between 1994 and 1996, Avon's sales grew 12 percent, to $4.8 billion, and Revlon's skyrocketed 25 percent, to $2.2 billion.

Then came a drug that would transform the anti-aging market forever: Botox. Derived from the deadly botulinum toxin, Botox was originally developed to treat a handful of rare muscle disorders. Then doctors discovered that it also smoothed wrinkles, literally paralyzing the facial muscles that make frown lines.

Injecting Botox seemed a drastic way to regain youth, but much to the surprise of the scientists who worked with the toxin, boomers loved it. Mitchell Brin first came across Botox in the early 1990s, when he was a young scientist at Columbia studying potential remedies for facial spasms. "We treated these patients, and what would happen is that the wrinkles on the treated side would go away," Brin recalled. Still, he couldn't imagine any company being able to sell it as a mass-market beauty treatment. "An anti-aging product looked very exciting, but it was an injection," Brin said. "That was scary at the time."

The manufacturer of Botox—Irvine, California–based Allergan—had won FDA approval in 1989 to market the toxin as a treatment for eyelid spasms and crossed eyes. Allergan hired Brin in 2000 to help further expand the market. Doctors were already using Botox off-label to treat everything from migraines to urinary incontinence. But Allergan's execs realized that the only way to make a real profit from Botox would be to sell it as a wrinkle eraser. Allergan started designing large-scale studies so it could win the FDA's blessing.

In 2002, the FDA approved Botox Cosmetic, and Allergan was utterly transformed. In the three years following the approval, Botox sales nearly doubled, to $831 million. By the end of the decade, the wildly popular injection would be a $1-billion-a-year blockbuster.

The success of Botox gave rise to a whole new category of products called "medical aesthetics." There were dermal fillers made of substances such as collagen, which could be injected into the face to tone down fine lines, and lasers to smooth out wrinkles, suck out cellulite, and even out skin color. Some of the world's largest companies embraced the term "anti-aging," including Johnson & Johnson, which partnered with start-ups to develop laser-based wrinkle removers and launched an anti-aging line of Neutrogena skin-care products.

Even though Allergan never marketed Botox using the term "anti-aging," its success surely gave Klatz and Goldman a boost. Botox made it acceptable for healthy people to get injections to preserve their youthfulness. The drug was so cool that doctors started holding "Botox parties," where groups of women would chitchat over cocktails while waiting their turn to get their wrinkles erased. Men started doing it, too. Suddenly getting a needle stick to stay young was in vogue. And it wasn't such a far cry from injecting poison to smooth out your face to shooting up hormones to restore your libido. Even the executives at Allergan recognized their role in creating a new industry—albeit one that they tried to disassociate themselves from. "I understand that people are experimenting with things like human growth hormone," Brin said. "I would have profound caution, until there are rigorous, controlled clinical trials, with the fine endpoints that are really going to establish efficacy."

Anti-aging clinics embraced Botox and all the other new tools wholeheartedly. Come get a prescription for HGH, some doctors promised, and we'll get rid of your wrinkles while you're here.

A4M's meteoric rise continued unabated, even as a string of legal mishaps cast serious doubts on its most famous pioneers. In 1995, the California Medical Board sanctioned Edmund Chein and put him on probation for, among other infractions, falsely claiming that he was an attorney. The *Los Angeles Times* reported that Chein's anti-aging clinic was distributing an article titled

"The NIA's Position on Growth Hormone Replacement Therapy in Adults," which erroneously stated that the federal National Institute on Aging had promoted the idea of giving growth hormone to healthy older people. In 2000, the California Medical Board tried to revoke Chein's license after alleging that he had improperly diagnosed a patient and then prescribed her growth hormone. The revocation was overturned.

In 2002, the California Medical Board charged Chein with 13 counts of negligence, incompetence, improper prescribing, inadequate record keeping, misconduct, dishonesty, and the unlawful dispensing of controlled substances. The 16-page accusation laid out the case of an unnamed patient who had sought treatment for emphysema at Chein's Palm Springs Life Extension Institute. Chein prescribed him testosterone, HGH, and other drugs, the complaint said. In 1999, Chein allegedly gave the patient HGH that had been mixed with insulin by two unlicensed employees in a back room at the anti-aging center. The patient suffered seizures and insulin shock. In 2005, Chein settled, agreeing to five years of probation, a $10,000 fine, and state monitoring.

Trouble also caught up with A4M founding physician Ward Dean. A West Point graduate and army flight surgeon, Dean had become fascinated with life extension long before he attended medical school. He served on the board of the American Aging Association, helped plan A4M's first gathering in Cancun, and actively recruited other physicians to the new organization. He might have achieved the same stature as Klatz and Goldman in anti-aging circles—were it not for the fact that he stopped paying his income taxes in 1997. Dean read a copy of the U.S. tax code, and he was positive that no one was legally obligated to pay taxes on income. "All of the other taxes had a specific code section that told clearly who was liable for a particular tax," he wrote on his Web site. "'Income Tax' was not even listed!"

In March 2005, the U.S. District Court for the Northern District of Florida indicted Dean for filing a collection of fake W-4s and 1040s that listed his taxable income from 1997 to 2002 as $0. (He had really earned $1.2 million during those years and owed $300,000 in taxes, according to court documents.) All together, Dean faced seven counts of tax evasion. In 2005, a jury convicted him on all counts, and he was sentenced to seven years in prison.

In a letter he wrote from the Federal Prison Camp in Atlanta four years later, Dean vowed to return to the anti-aging world after his release in June 2012. "I'll probably continue as the Medical Director of Vitamin Research Products in Carson City, Nevada," Dean wrote. "Prior to my trial, I was also working with International Anti-Aging Systems, in the United Kingdom, to develop a very sophisticated aging measurement system." He planned to keep his distance from A4M, however. His major gripe about the organization's approach to anti-aging, said the prisoner, was its "over-commercialization of the concept, prior to the proper scientific foundation having been laid." Still, he added, "I have to give Drs. Klatz and Goldman a lot of credit for popularizing the concept of anti-aging medicine."

Turney, the HGH connoisseur who started the El Dorado longevity spa in Mexico, injected the hormone for the next 14 years, but not at El Dorado. Less than two years after it opened, Turney grew fed up with Mexican politics and abandoned the clinic. "The governor, the mayor, the police chief started coming for *mordidas*—payoffs," Turney said. "So I took the list of patients and split them up among 26 doctors in the United States who wanted to do this. We coined a protocol, 'adult pituitary deficiency,' and they still use that to justify prescriptions to aging people. It's viable. I think it's very viable."

In 1995, Turney legally changed his name to Lazarus Long, the name of a recurring character in books written by Robert A. Heinlein, a libertarian science fiction writer. Heinlein's stories championed self-reliance and individual thinking—not to mention the fantastical idea that people could live forever. The fictional Long partook of a rejuvenation treatment made from blood grown in test tubes. He was 224 years old and defying death at every turn. "I always identified with the character," Turney said. "I checked Internet phone books all over the world. I could find only one other Lazarus Long, and he was in Australia. I thought why not?"

Turney stopped injecting HGH when concerns over illegal doping in sports led many doctors to stop prescribing the hormone. Then he tried to start his own country called New Utopia, located on a 400-square-mile island 160 miles west of Grand Cayman Island. "I'm building the Venice of the Caribbean," he said. "Instead of roads it will be waterways. Instead of cars it will be gondolas and water taxis. There will be a big medical center with a whole wing for anti-aging medicine." New Utopia would be a principality with no taxes and no real government, and he would call himself Prince Lazarus, Turney said. "The intrusiveness of government has always been a problem for me," he added.

Turney hoped someday to start taking HGH again. "If I can do it without causing grief to anybody, I'd like to get back on it. Not here. In New Utopia."

In 1999, the Securities and Exchange Commission (SEC) accused Turney of selling $350 million in unregistered bonds to fund New Utopia. He spent ten months trying to prove to the

SEC that even though he had written on his Web site that he was considering a bond offering, he had not actually issued any bonds. In 2000, the SEC issued an injunction alleging Turney had raised $24,000, but it waived all penalties based on his inability to pay. A decade later he was still trying to raise money for the project. But he was confident that his utilitarian dream would come true and that it would provide a home for fellow HGH enthusiasts.

Where other anti-aging pioneers went astray, Klatz and Goldman forged ahead. On his résumé, Klatz listed patents he had secured for a handful of medical devices he had invented, including a brain-cooling instrument and a gizmo meant to improve blood circulation. There was no indication, however, that the products ever made it to market. Klatz also boasted about being named a "top 10 medical innovator in biomedical technology" by the National Institute of Electromedical Information. But the Web site of this nonprofit "institute" gave very little insight as to its credentials.

Goldman, too, seemed prone to self-importance. Among achievements he listed on his résumé was that he had served "as an affiliate at the Philosophy of Education Research Center, Graduate School of Education, Harvard University." According to Harvard, affiliates weren't teachers or researchers. Rather, they were ordinary people invited to attend public presentations and sometimes to lecture on "topics of interest." But to the unfortunate laypeople placing their trust in these pioneers of anti-aging medicine, the mere mention of Harvard might be enough to make Goldman look like academic royalty. Goldman also wrote that he was "the recipient of the Gold Medal for Science, the Grand Prize for Medicine, the Humanitarian Award, and the Business Development Award." From where, though?

Klatz and Goldman held an annual conference in Las Vegas, Nevada, which they christened the World Congress on Anti-Aging Medicine. In the early days of A4M, the World Congress was a lowbrow affair held in a circus tent, which was pitched between two buildings at a hotel off the Strip. But as the organization grew richer, Klatz and Goldman moved their flagship event to the ritzy Venetian Hotel, a palatial 36-story casino on the strip, where every guest room was a luxury suite with a sunken living room, a dining nook, and remote-controlled Roman blinds.

Despite its overinflated title, the World Congress—at least the exposition—appeared little more than a hormone trade show, where hundreds of distributors touted their hormone-packaging services. A cavernous exhibit hall housed up to 400 companies, each of which paid up to $15,000 for a booth to display its wares.

A4M points out that its expositions are separate from its educational conferences. Exhibitors are invited on a first-come first-served basis, and A4M does not vouch for any of the products or services on display. Not surprising since the expositions became a magnet for all manner of snake-oil salesmen pushing anti-aging cure-alls. Tooth-whitening products and multivitamins shared the floor with the likes of the Cellubike, an exercise bike with infrared lights that purportedly erased unsightly cellulite. "Hi, have you ever had a colon cleanse?" shouted an exhibitor cheerfully to convention attendees sauntering through the exhibit hall one year. His company was pitching a $10,000 machine that flushed out colons, purportedly so they wouldn't become breeding grounds for polyps and cancer. A colon cleanse could even shave those unwanted love handles, the exhibitor said, as he held up a photo of what one could only assume was a happily cleaned-out patient. "He lost 12 pounds. He had a big ol' gut before."

The Las Vegas extravaganza also drew legions of doctors who were curious to learn about this new branch of medicine. Klatz and Goldman trotted out the Rudman research and other papers on hormones, and they recruited guest lecturers to talk about hormone replacement. A4M's membership ranks had grown to 7,000 by 2000. Five years later, the organization had 11,500 followers, and at the end of the decade it boasted 20,000 physician members in 100 countries. By that time, A4M was staging 30 conferences a year all over the world, from Bangkok and Shanghai to Melbourne and Mexico City. At each event, devotees greeted Klatz and Goldman as gurus of this new brand of medicine.

But their theories were still dismissed by mainstream scientists, so Klatz and Goldman found new ways to get the message out. They published new medical journals, some of which seemed devoid of rigorous scientific review. In volume 10 of A4M's journal *Anti-Aging Therapeutics*, for example, a doctor named Patrick Hanaway wrote a paper describing how to personalize hormone treatments. The article suggested a regimen of tests to figure out how best to prescribe HGH and other hormones to each patient. "Hormonal assessments, based upon this 3-dimensional perspective of urine, serum, and saliva, will help generate the best answers in meeting the needs of each individual patient," he wrote. Hanaway happened to be the chief medical officer of Genova Diagnostics, a company that sold more than 125 different medical tests.

A4M combined commerce with education. The organization staged continuing medical education (CME) courses, which awarded credits that doctors could use to maintain their licenses. The Las Vegas conference doled out dozens of CME credits. And in 2004, A4M launched a fellowship program, which issued its graduates certificates in anti-aging medicine.

Doctors simply had to complete eight modules—weekend seminars taught by other anti-aging doctors at swank hotels like the Bahia Mar Beach Resort & Yachting Center in Fort Lauderdale, Florida. A4M advertised the program as the equivalent of a board certification in a legitimate medical specialty. Even Klatz and Goldman claimed on their résumés to be "board certified" in anti-aging medicine.

But there was no such board certification. Real medical specialties had to be approved by the American Medical Association Council on Medical Education and the American Board of Medical Specialties—neither of which recognized anti-aging as appropriate for certification. Those organizations' written guidelines required that "the emergence of a new medical specialty must be based on a substantial advancement in medical science and represent a distinct and well-defined field of medical practice." They also demanded that anyone tasked with certifying doctors must be free of conflicts of interest. Since it looked like A4M's members themselves would stand to profit from the growth of the specialty they invented, it seemed like a long shot that anti-aging would ever be approved as a recognized medical specialty. A spokeswoman for the American Board of Medical Specialties said her organization once got a call from A4M but never a formal application. "They may have realized they couldn't meet the requirements," she said.

A4M did not explain why it believes the term "board certified" is accurate, but it stated that "of approximately 270 specialist medical societies and medical boards, only 24 . . . in total have been approved by the American Board of Medical Specialties."

Many doctors, following their leaders Klatz and Goldman, promoted themselves as "board certified" in anti-aging medicine nonetheless. In 2005, the Texas Medical Board fined Lane Sebring $500 for placing ads that used the phrase "board certified in anti-aging medicine." Two years later, it levied a $250 fine on Theodore Piliszek for the same violation. And after San Diego doctor Robert Sterner was caught improperly prescribing marijuana in an undercover sting, the California Medical Board set out to revoke his license. Sterner "mistakenly believed he was properly certified by the American Board of Anti-Aging Medicine," according to court papers. Sterner was put on probation for seven years. He stopped referring to himself as board certified in anti-aging.

But whenever one anti-aging doctor stumbled, another three or four popped up to fill the demand for hormones. And they had no trouble finding patients like Howard Turney, who, like his idol Lazarus Long, would do anything to stay young. At 78, many years after his El Dorado adventure had ended, Turney felt good enough to play racquetball for an hour each day. But he craved the HGH that had sharpened up his eyesight and made his hand stop shaking. He only wanted a little bit, he said—not enough to endanger his health. "Lemonade can be dangerous if you drink too much too quickly. Anything can be dangerous if you overdo it. Lemonade in moderate amounts is good for you. It's the same way with growth hormone," Turney said.

Behind every Howard-Turney-turned-Lazarus-Long were thousands more people who were completely won over by the anti-aging hoopla. Some dabbled in one or two supplements for a short time; others embraced extreme hormone replacement as a lifelong regimen. But the sheer ignorance these patients had about the substances they were ingesting could seriously harm them. Misinformation could prove to be the poison that tainted the fountain of youth.

CHAPTER 2

All for Money

Ron Rothenberg was the tenth doctor to earn A4M's certification, and one of the most sought-after anti-aging specialists in youth-obsessed Southern California. On a warm March day in 2006, he burst through the door of his San Diego clinic, a cell phone pressed to his ear. His nurse prepped him for the busy day ahead. He would have in-depth consultations with three new patients and follow-up meetings with several more. Rothenberg's impressive pedigree added to his allure: The Columbia University–trained M.D.'s center, called the California Healthspan Institute, was based on the campus of renowned Scripps Memorial Hospital, where Rothenberg still did occasional stints in the emergency room. But anti-aging was his true passion. "Wind me up," he said, while rattling off the life-extending benefits of hormones during a meeting with a new patient. "The problem is stopping me, because I'm so excited about this."

During a break from meeting all his new patients, Rothenberg caught up with Howard Benedict, a retired dentist he had met while surfing in Cabo San Lucas, Mexico, in 1999. Arthritis had forced Benedict into retirement. Rothenberg put him on a $10,000-a-year regimen of HGH, testosterone, and 30 vitamins and supplements. Benedict's pain eased so much he could ride his bike and surf for hours at a stretch, he reported. "Those other guys my age, they're only out there surfing for a half-hour," said the 61-year-old Benedict, a strapping, mustachioed fellow with a full head of white hair. "Both my brothers are totally bald, and they have these big pot bellies. They have so many physical problems. I don't have any. I feel good all over." A sly smile crept across his face. "I feel like I'm 20 years old with my wife. It's just amazing."

Rothenberg chimed in, "Your youthful hormone levels help. If you get an X-ray, you'll still see arthritis. But you've improved your quality of life. I see that every day."

Treatment plans such as Benedict's, Rothenberg said, were designed to guarantee "rectangularization," a concept that Rothenberg explained with a smile and a flourish of hand gestures. "Stay strong and healthy to the end," he said, "then fall off a cliff fast." Anti-aging proponents preferred that route to "triangularization," or the slow descent toward death that their parents had suffered. "Rather than spending a few years in the ICU or a nursing home, why not fall apart fast and die?" Rothenberg asked enthusiastically.

A4M doctors insisted they were not guaranteeing their patients would live longer; they were merely promising them a better quality of life. But Rothenberg, an endlessly cheerful man with more than a passing resemblance to the comic actor Gene Wilder, wasn't shy about assuring patients he could actually extend their lives. "We anticipate that with HGH replacement along with other indicated hormone replacement including nutrition and exercise we can now expect to live to the age of 125 in excellent health," he wrote on the Web site of his California Healthspan Institute (www.ehealthspan.com).

Rothenberg put all his new patients through an intense workup. Several weeks before their first appointment, he sent them a 34-page "wellness and lifestyle assessment." They had to answer questions about every medical problem they and all their family members had ever suffered, and they had to list every food they had eaten in the previous two days. They were asked to describe their exercise routines in detail and to rate the frequency with which they experienced a number of symptoms ("pain in left side under rib cage," "calf muscle cramps while walking," "sensitivity to cold temperatures," "wake up in the middle of the night craving sweets," and so forth). And they had to detail their psychological health, stress level at work, and even their religious practices. To develop the most individualized anti-aging routine, Rothenberg explained, "we have to look everywhere."

All of Rothenberg's new patients were sent saliva-testing kits, which he said he could use to measure their hormone levels. Patients spit into vials four times in a single day, then shipped the samples off to a lab, which tested them for testosterone, progesterone, estrogen, and other hormones. Then patients were directed to diagnostic centers, where they rolled up their sleeves and gave multiple vials of blood. The samples were tested for everything from calcium and sodium levels to thyroid and liver function. One of the blood tests measured insulin-like growth factor (IGF-1), which is produced in response to growth hormone. Anti-aging doctors scrutinized IGF-1 levels to determine which patients should get prescriptions for HGH injections.

But there was more. Rothenberg also sent patients off to be evaluated by an exercise physiologist and to consult with his in-house nutritionist on how to improve their diets. Rothenberg chatted with new patients for at least an hour apiece, advising them on how to take all the hormones and vitamins he was pre-scribing and how to incorporate them into a total program of improved diet and fitness. Each patient received a fat binder full of instructions and menus. Total cost: more than $2,000, not in-cluding follow-up visits. And because insurance companies did-n't recognize aging as a disease—and most didn't endorse saliva testing, either—patients shouldered the bulk of the expenses.

Like most anti-aging doctors, Rothenberg was his own pa-tient. He had been drawn to hormone therapy in 1997, when he was 51 and working in emergency medicine. "I was losing my edge in subtle ways," he recalled. "I was losing my memory. I was trying to go to the gym, but things weren't working somehow. Libido-wise, it was take it or leave it." He dropped in on A4M's second Las Vegas conference and was instantly hooked. "Here was this endless world of new things to learn about," Rothenberg said. He started trying anti-aging therapies himself. "I went from one hormone to the next. I needed growth hormone," he said. "It's OK to experiment on and off, to get a feel for what it's doing." Over time, he also began in-jecting himself with testosterone, taking thyroid hormone, and swallowing a daily assortment of vitamins.

The propensity of anti-aging doctors to partake of the very therapies they were prescribing made it that much easier for them to convince patients that all those hormones and supple-ments were safe. After all, if your own doctor is taking HGH, how dangerous can it possibly be? Rothenberg played up his

virility by filling his office with photographs of himself surfing. He hung a surfboard over his desk as a testament to his
own youthful spirit.

New doctors drawn into A4M's ranks seemed totally persuaded—not just by the notion that they could keep themselves and their patients young, but also by the irresistible
opportunity to escape the shackles of managed care. Anti-
aging was a cash business, so doctors could operate completely
off the radar of Medicare and private insurers. They didn't have
to fill out reams of claims forms or bicker with insurance ex-
aminers over shrinking reimbursement rates. And they didn't
have to cram in 30 patients a day just to make ends meet. Instead, they could spend hours with a handful of patients, tailoring hormone regimens to fit those patients' individual
needs and taking time to listen to all the details of their aches
and pains. "We don't deal with insurance. That's the luxury of
this," Rothenberg said one evening, while dining on sushi at a
trendy restaurant near his clinic. "It's like the personal family
doctor from the Norman Rockwell era."

The undying trust that patients had in this new branch of
medicine seemed to allow anti-aging doctors to stack on high-
priced services and treatments. Some of the treatments were
purely cosmetic. When Allergan started teaching physicians
how to inject Botox to treat wrinkles, anti-aging doctors clam-
ored to sign up for the training—a trend that didn't surprise
Allergan CEO David Pyott. Like most anti-aging medications,
the cosmetic form of Botox wasn't reimbursed by insurance
companies, and that was a plus for the A4M crowd. "What they
see is escape from Alcatraz," Pyott said. "How can I get away
from insurance companies making my life miserable? How

can I get away from the phone calls, the denial of coverage? People have been lining up to say, 'How do I learn Botox?'"

Not all the services anti-aging doctors offered were as transparently effective as Botox, however. During their first consultation with Rothenberg, patients were escorted into a small room in the back of his clinic and hooked up to a machine called the H-Scan. The computerized testing equipment included a Breathalyzer-like device and a panel of six buttons with flashing red lights. One H-Scan session, which cost $105, was designed to measure memory, lung capacity, reaction time, hearing, sensitivity to touch, and other so-called biomarkers of aging. During the memory test, the device's buttons flashed in random sequences. Patients were asked to remember the illuminations in the correct sequence and press the buttons corresponding to the pattern. The computer added another button to each round to boost the difficulty—2, 3, 6; then 2, 3, 6, 1; then 2, 3, 6, 1, 3, and so on. At the end of the test, H-Scan told patients their "biological age"—their real age, as measured by how well their body was actually functioning, rather than by the number of years they'd been on earth.

Richard Hochschild, who developed the H-Scan, was the first to admit that the test was somewhat limited in its ability to reveal much about how well people were aging. "Your biological age could depend on a thousand different things. We picked 12," said Hochschild, who lived a short freeway drive from Rothenberg in Corona del Mar, California. Hochschild worried that the whole business of managing the aging process had become, well, too much of a business—a suspicion that was strengthened by his few visits to A4M's conferences. "When I go, I don't hear a lot of science," he said. "I do hear a lot of marketing."

Rothenberg's patients may not have questioned his high-priced tests and therapies, however. One 52-year-old woman reported rather nonchalantly that she was taking 48 supplement pills a day, plus estrogen in skin creams and injections, all of which Rothenberg had prescribed. She bragged that her real age, according to the H-Scan, was 40, and she was certain that if she were to take it again, she would improve her score. "I keep getting better and younger," she said. Such positive feedback from patients probably reassured Rothenberg that his therapies worked. "Where's the big double-blind study, placebo controlled? It's never going to happen," he said. "Let's take our best shot now."

More and more doctors followed Rothenberg's lead and joined A4M. They came from emergency medicine and family practice, from gynecology and geriatrics. They packed the exhibit halls at A4M's conferences and signed up for the fellowship in droves. Many took courses from Rothenberg himself, who became one of A4M's most popular faculty members.

But these eager students were learning about hormones from people who may not have been the best qualified to be teaching them. Klatz, Goldman, Rothenberg, and others who trained anti-aging doctors were not certified endocrinologists, doctors who specialize in the study of hormones. In fact, anti-aging medicine attracted very few endocrinologists, because most of those hormone docs believed there were flaws in the premise that people could stop the clock by restoring their hormones to youthful levels. "It's invalid and it's misleading," said Mary Lee Vance, an endocrinologist and professor of medicine for the University of Virginia Health System. Vance sometimes consulted for the U.S. Department of Justice (DOJ) and the U.S. Drug Enforcement Agency (DEA) on cases involving HGH, and she was horrified to see how freely anti-aging doctors were pre-scribing the hormone to patients who didn't need it. "They're in it for the money," Vance said. "That really offends my sensi-bilities."

Vance inadvertently fueled the anti-aging craze in 1990, when she wrote an editorial to accompany Daniel Rudman's original *New England Journal* paper about HGH in older men. She wrote that his research "should be viewed as an important beginning." They were words she would live to regret. What Vance meant was that scientists should perform more studies to determine the true benefits and risks of giving growth hor-mone to healthy people. What anti-aging entrepreneurs read was entirely different. As far as they were concerned, a re-spected endocrinologist was telling them to prescribe the hor-mone to cure aging. "It's misuse," Vance said. "It's totally wrong."

And it was unlikely patients fully understood that Rud-man's own research suggested that prescribing HGH to healthy adults was a bad idea. In 1993, Rudman copublished an 18-month study of HGH in 83 healthy men. It was a much larger cohort than what he had looked at for his flagship paper, and he observed them for a longer period of time. During that second study, several men suffered adverse reactions, such as carpal tunnel syndrome, enlarged breasts, and high blood sugar. All told, 29 men ended up dropping out of the study. The report—complete with details about the side effects—attracted considerably less fanfare than the famous 1990 study, because it was published in the relatively obscure British jour-nal *Clinical Endocrinology*.

In 2003, disturbed by the proliferation of anti-aging clinics and Web sites, the editors of the *New England Journal* posted the first Rudman paper online, along with a stark warning. "This article has been cited in potentially misleading e-mail advertisements," they wrote. They went on to explain that they were taking the unusual step of offering the original article for free, along with several others laying out the perils of prescribing HGH to healthy adults. They cited a cautionary line from Vance's original editorial: "Because there are so many unanswered questions about the use of growth hormone in the elderly and in adults with growth hormone deficiency, its general use now or in the immediate future is not justified."

Vance included in the package a new editorial titled "Can Growth Hormone Prevent Aging?" She cited studies that were more rigorous than the Rudman research and that called into question the wisdom of HGH therapy. One trial—which, unlike Rudman's, included women and was double-blind and placebo-controlled—showed that even though HGH improved body composition, it did not increase muscle strength. In fact, HGH could cause water retention, which could easily be mistaken for an increase in nonfatty body mass. But that didn't mean the muscles had grown stronger. In another study, a group of aging men did ten weeks of strength training and took either a placebo or HGH. Adding growth hormone did nothing to increase their muscle power. "Going to the gym is beneficial," Vance concluded, "and certainly cheaper than growth hormone."

The biggest worry was that growth hormone might raise the risk of cancer. It was a valid concern. HGH, after all, promotes growth, and many doctors suspected that tiny, undetectable malignancies might balloon in the presence of a potent stimulator. Experiments mixing cancer cells with HGH in test tubes confirmed that there was reason to fret. But scientists would never be able to prove the theory in humans because it would be unethical to expose healthy people to any therapy suspected of causing cancer. Furthermore, because cancer is more prevalent in older people to begin with, it would be difficult to determine if HGH was the true instigator.

But there was plenty of evidence to warrant caution. A 1998 study of 304 healthy men found that the risk of developing prostate cancer was significantly higher in people who had naturally high levels of IGF-1 in their blood. In more than 300 studies, people who were very tall—suggesting their bodies made more growth hormone than average—had a 20 percent or higher risk of developing breast, prostate, or colon cancer than did people of normal stature. And there was a prevalence of colon cancer among patients with acromegaly, a disease caused by abnormally high levels of growth hormone and marked by the excessive growth of hands, feet, and other extremities.

The anecdotal evidence against HGH was equally disturbing. In 2008, a group of endocrinologists at Cedars-Sinai Medical Center in Los Angeles published a case study about a 68-year-old who had been taking HGH for anti-aging purposes for seven years before he developed colon cancer. He had the intestinal disorder Crohn's disease, which put him at increased risk for cancer in the first place, so the scientists had no way of determining whether HGH was the actual culprit. Still, said Shlomo Melmed, coauthor of the study and dean of the hospital's medical faculty, "what is known is that once a tumor is initiated, HGH can exacerbate its growth."

Another case was that of Hanneke Hops, a northern California woman who told the *San Francisco Chronicle* in 2003 that daily injections of HGH were making her strong and healthy enough to run marathons, ride horses, and fly planes. Three months later she died from cancer, her liver riddled with inoperable tumors. Her son, Erick Schenkhuizen, told the paper in 2006 that he believed her treatments had fed an undiscovered malignancy. "If she hadn't taken the hormones, she could still be alive today," he said.

When Rothenberg trained other doctors in prescribing HGH, he sometimes told them that the hormone was unlikely to cause cancer survivors to relapse, and he referred to a study coauthored by Vance. But the patients in Vance's study had severe HGH deficiencies and were given only tiny doses of the hormone.

Vance was incensed to learn that anti-aging advocates were quoting such a limited experiment as proof that HGH doesn't cause cancer, especially when other research demonstrated it might. "They're misquoting [scientific] literature up the wazoo," she said. At the time, Rothenberg responded by pointing to three other studies he said supported his viewpoint. "There is no increase in cancer rates when growth hormone replacement therapy is utilized," he said. "This has been extensively reviewed in the medical literature."

The anti-aging crowd's tendency to skirt science even caused consternation within its own ranks. In 2002, more than 50 scientists—including some former A4M supporters—signed a paper called "Position Statement on Human Aging," which was published in *Scientific American* and the *Journal of Gerontology*. The article started with this declaration about the anti-aging industry: "The products being sold have no scientifically demonstrated efficacy, in some cases they may be harmful, and those selling them often misrepresent the science upon which they are based."

A year later, at the 2003 Las Vegas conference, the event's longtime producer, Primedia, announced that it would ditch A4M and instead put on a competing event focused entirely on the science of longevity. A4M member and UCLA scientist L. Stephen Coles had signed the position statement and planned to join the dissenting organization. At A4M's conference, he walked up to the podium and declared that there was no such thing as anti-aging medicine. The crowd howled. In recalling the split several years later, Coles said, "Several companies and private practices were built on the idea that replacing growth hormone was the secret to anti-aging medicine. This fantasy lasted a long time. But it has proven to be a delusion."

After Coles spoke, Klatz went on the stage and criticized him and others for signing the *Journal of Gerontology* article. The incident was recounted in detail in the book *Healthy Aging*, by famed natural-medicine doctor Andrew Weil, who attended that year's A4M conference out of sheer curiosity. Klatz asked audience members how many of them used HGH in their practices. Hands shot up all over the room, Weil recalled. Klatz told them anyone could live past 100, and he got a standing ovation. Weil never attended another A4M conference. "They want anti-aging to be a recognized specialty," Weil said. "To have doctors selling it makes it seem official. But I don't think it's a legitimate field. It's dangerous and exploitative."

A4M, in turn, has accused Weil of engaging in highly commercial activities based on the same concepts that Weil said were not legitimate. Weil's opinion was also tainted, according to A4M, because he had lectured for a direct competitor of A4M.

Klatz flatly denied the *Journal of Gerontology*'s position, too. As Weil reported in *Healthy Aging*, Klatz wrote in boldface type in a letter to A4M's members: "A premeditated, malicious, and deliberate disinformation campaign directed at dismantling the single most unified group of innovative physicians and scientists in America is now underway. A powerful old-boy network is investing enormous time, personnel, and financial resources on destroying today's most successful, most popular, and fastest growing medical society."

In 2006, Primedia got out of the conference business altogether. A4M refugees Rick Merner and Greg Fillmore wanted to keep the competing event going, so they formed a new organization, Age Management Medicine Group (AMMG). The group held conferences in Nevada and Florida, often just a week or so after A4M's events in those cities. AMMG members openly criticized Klatz and Goldman for selling out. "There were a lot of charlatans that paid Klatz and Goldman for a speaking slot," said Coles, who had particularly strong views. "They were salespeople cloaked as scientific experts. Whatever company could pay for booth space was brought in, as long as their check didn't bounce." A4M's response to Coles's criticism was that "his comments are ridiculous and that of a very weak and unsuccessful business competitor."

A4M's commercialism led some critics to nickname the organization "all for money," although A4M claimed that it maintained "no commercial interests or biases in the [anti-aging] industry."

AMMG's conferences were considerably less flashy than A4M's—the exhibit hall filled just two rows in a tiny room. But AMMG needed money too, and it took sponsorship funding from Cenegenics, one of the biggest chains of anti-aging clinics in the United States. When Cenegenics's chief medical officer, Jeffry Life, presented a lecture on growth hormone at the 2009 conference—a talk that attendees could count toward continuing medical education credits—he flipped through slides labeled with the Cenegenics logo.

Such mixing of education and advertising bothered people like Gregory Petersburg, who had fled A4M to escape its commercialism. Petersburg bought a booth at an AMMG conference to exhibit his office-management products for anti-aging doctors. But he was disappointed. "From an ethical standpoint, I don't think a sponsoring organization should be selecting the speakers," Petersburg said.

Despite the competition from AMMG, most of A4M's members stayed loyal to Klatz and Goldman. The anti-aging trailblazers continued to vilify anyone who dared to criticize them publicly, and defamation suits appeared to be their weapon of choice. Around the time of the AMMG split, Klatz and Goldman were waging war against two of the most well-known scholars in the field of aging: S. Jay Olshansky, a professor at the University of Illinois School of Public Health, and Thomas Perls, a professor at Boston University School of Medicine. Klatz and Goldman had filed a defamation suit against the academics in 2004. They alleged that Olshansky "engaged in a fraudulent campaign here in the United States and internationally to destroy A4M, to destroy the reputation of Goldman and Klatz, and to destroy the business developed by Goldman and Klatz." Perls, they charged, joined in later. And as a result of "defamatory statements and tortious interference," the suit said, A4M lost at least $50 million worth of business.

Olshansky and Perls believed that what they were doing was warning the public about what they regarded as illicit prescribing of HGH for anti-aging. In 2001, they participated in a workshop titled "Is There an 'Anti-Aging' Medicine?" which was sponsored by the International Longevity Center (ILC) in New

York. Among the workshop's findings, which the ILC published and circulated, were studies proving that mice that overproduced growth hormone didn't live as long as normal mice, and mice that didn't make enough growth hormone, or just didn't respond to it, actually lived longer than average. Such findings led the team to warn that "efforts to restore circulating growth hormone to youthful levels in older individuals may be misguided." Olshansky led the group of scientists who wrote the position statement that was published in the *Journal of Gerontology*. And in 2004, he and Perls cowrote a paper for a special edition of the same journal called "Anti-Aging Medicine: The Hype and the Reality." They pulled no punches in their conclusion: "Our advice regarding alleged anti-aging interventions is simple—*caveat emptor.*"

Olshansky had more than just a passing interest in HGH. After his son was diagnosed with growth hormone deficiency, Olshansky set out to learn everything he could about HGH. "He had a malformed pituitary gland, which was documented with an MRI," Olshansky said. "So his was a known, recognized condition for which growth hormone is legal." Olshansky scoured all the research on HGH and even recruited his students to study the drug too, so he could prepare for any side effects his son might encounter. The studies showed some risk of diabetes and colon cancer, which Olshansky deemed manageable with careful screening throughout his son's life. But Olshansky was struck by how few studies had been done on HGH in grown-ups. "If you ask these anti-aging people about the scientific literature on growth hormone, they say, 'Oh, there have been thousands of studies. It's one of the most extensively studied hormones.' Well, yeah—in children," Olshansky said. "But not in healthy adults, and that's who they're giving it to. You can't extrapolate from children to healthy adults."

A4M completely rejected Olshansky's opinion, stating, "Mr. Olshansky is not a clinician or physician, nor is he a biologist or biological researcher; he is a statistician who lacks clinical acumen. His willingness to say or do anything to promote his position is well known. The clinical literature is rife with reports of excellent clinical results in both adults and children from the judicious and appropriate use of HGH for replacement purposes, in laboratory confirmed cases of deficiency, which is precisely the method which A4M and its member physicians has always endorsed." A4M offered a list of 21 articles that it said supported its position.

In 2002, Olshansky inaugurated a mock awards program called the Silver Fleece, which was designed to expose the most outrageous claims about slowing or reversing aging. The award, a bottle of vegetable oil labeled "Snake Oil," went to A4M. Two years later, Olshansky presented the Silver Fleece to A4M's *International Journal of Anti-Aging Medicine* and to Market America, a company that had partnered with Klatz and Goldman to develop anti-aging remedies. Olshansky blasted them for selling a suite of dietary supplements called Prime Blends, which they claimed would prompt the body to pump out more HGH naturally. "Market America uses clever hype and pseudo-scientific mumbo-jumbo to convince consumers that 'nutraceuticals' and 'cosmeceuticals' can alter the aging process," Olshansky said in a press release announcing the faux award. "About the only thing these anti-aging products do is fatten the wallets of those selling them."

In their lawsuit, Klatz and Goldman alleged that Olshansky conducted a "modern-day witch hunt" against A4M. In 2003, they alleged, Olshansky went to the Las Vegas conference and denounced A4M to, among others, the executive vice president of Market America. Olshansky allegedly told the Market America executive that the products were "unproven" and "virtually useless," and he called Klatz and Goldman "quacks" and an "embarrassment to the scientific community." Market America later pulled out of its contract with Klatz and Goldman.

According to A4M, "The 'Silver Fleece award' was a media-garnering stunt concocted by Mr. Olshansky, who is not a trained physician and has no medical or surgical training in aging intervention. This stunt was part of an elaborate and larger campaign of disparagement by Mr. Olshansky and Dr. Perls, aimed at discrediting A4M and its founders, Dr. Goldman and Dr. Klatz, in order to advance their own business agenda in promoting their own anti-aging projects and anti-aging conferences, sponsored by competitor entities to A4M, at which Mr. Olshansky and/or Dr. Perls themselves were featured speakers, or personally assisted with the conference organizer's programs."

Perls, a geriatrician at Boston Medical Center, happened upon anti-aging medicine during his own research on centenarians. In 1994, Perls founded the New England Centenarian Study and began interviewing people over 100 who lived in eight suburbs of Boston. Perls and his team studied everything from the genetics to the family histories of their long-lived subjects. And as they began to publish their research, A4M types took notice. "I was finding my work quoted by these characters who were saying they could stop and reverse aging," Perls said. He went to A4M's Web site and was flabbergasted by what he found. "They had this very pernicious view of elderly people. They had pictures of old people sitting in wheelchairs and staring at nursing home walls, and they were saying, 'This is aging. This is what getting old is all about.'" Perls was more than happy to join Olshansky's crusade against anti-aging medicine.

In 2005, as lawyers from Olshansky's and Perls's respective universities were fighting the A4M suit, the professors tried to bring attention to the rampant off-label use of HGH. In October 2005, they published an article in the *Journal of the American Medical Association* titled "Provision or Distribution of Growth Hormone for 'Antiaging': Clinical and Legal Issues." It urged federal and state agencies to devote more resources to tracking down physicians who were illegally prescribing HGH off-label for anti-aging purposes. "Given the clinical concerns and the legal issues involved, we believe that physicians or other persons who currently market, distribute, or administer GH to their patients for any reason other than the well-defined approved (ie, legal) uses of the drug, should not do so," they wrote. They implored the FDA and medical organizations to educate the public about the legal and medical risks of using growth hormone. "There's evidence that growth hormone accelerates aging and increases the risk for age-related diseases," Perls said. "In studies, it shortens lifespan. That's really the outrageous paradox here. It has the opposite effect of the claims."

At first, Klatz and Goldman were determined to fight their defamation suit all the way through to a jury trial, and they demanded damages of $300 million. So lawyers for Olshansky and Perls began gathering evidence against A4M and its supporters. "My university came right to the rescue," Olshansky recalled. "They said, 'Jay, don't worry about a thing. You're doing what you're supposed to be doing—you're protecting public health.'" But Olshansky was curious, so he sat in on a deposition regarding one of the products that Klatz and Goldman were promoting. "They said they had scientific evidence to support it, including an article that was published. So we deposed the first author of that article," Olshansky said, referring to a scientist whose identity was sealed along with all the documents related to the case. The scientist was grilled so ruthlessly, Olshansky said, that in his view, the process may have caused A4M's lawyers to request a settlement.

A4M had good reason to resolve the suit as quickly as possible. Tarsus Group, an international media conglomerate based in the United Kingdom, had taken an interest in A4M's conference business. This type of lawsuit might be unbecoming of Tarsus, a multimillion-dollar company that was publicly traded on the London stock exchange. In November 2006, Tarsus shelled out $60 million to acquire an 80 percent stake in the conference. That same month, A4M settled with Olshansky and Perls. No money changed hands, though all the parties in the Perls settlement agreed that they wouldn't say anything bad about each other for two years.

Olshansky was relieved—and a little disappointed. "I actually wanted it to go to trial," he said. "I wanted to see them testify under oath, and I wanted us to speak openly without worrying about somebody trying to suppress what we were saying. That lawsuit was all about suppression. It was all about stopping us from speaking our minds. And it did not work."

Exactly two years after the settlement, Perls launched a Web site called Growth Hormone/HGH/Antiaging and Sports (www .hghwatch.com) and turned it into an exhaustive collection of articles designed to expose A4M's flaws. The home page shouted the site's mission: "The real truth about Growth Hormone for Anti-Aging and Sports. It's Quackery and Hucksterism." Perls collected scientific studies on human growth hormone and posted details about them in a section he called "Shortens life span!" One of the studies he described, published in 2002 by the

National Institute on Aging, examined the use of growth hormone in healthy men and women. Although some participants saw an increase in lean body mass and a decrease in fat, 40 percent reported side effects such as joint pain, swelling, and glucose intolerance. The scientists said that there was no conclusive proof that HGH prevents aging, and any patients considering taking it should heed warnings about adverse effects. They noted previous research suggesting that long-term treatment with HGH might increase the risk of cancer.

A4M responded to Perls's charges as follows: "By opening a website, Dr. Perls has made the campaign of disinformation regarding HGH replacement therapy a career activity. He likely reaps notoriety as well as monetary compensation as a consultant by engaging in this activity, thus his motivations and claims should be considered carefully. The website's 'What is the law' page (http://www.hghwatch.com/whatisthelaw.html) gives misleading and incomplete explanation of 21 U.S.C. § 333(e), a provision of the Food, Drug, and Cosmetic Act (FDCA)." A4M also stated, "The focus of lawmakers and Congress has always been to address non-medical use, i.e., improper use by competitive elite athletes, sports people and teenagers. When [the regulation] was written, there were no anti-aging doctors or profession in existence. In fact, the anti-aging medical profession did not even exist until 5 years after the 1988 statute was enacted."

Perls, like Olshansky, was disappointed that he missed the chance to fight A4M in front of a judge and jury. But as he reminisced about the suit in his suburban Boston home, bustling with three children and four dogs, he conceded that settling was the right thing to do to shield his wife and family from the nuttiness of A4M. "They didn't care about it like I did—they just wanted me out," he said. "If I had been single, I could have taken [Klatz and Goldman] to the mattress. It would have been an opportunity to take them down."

A4M's 2008 Las Vegas conference started just a few weeks after Perls's anti-HGH site went up. But physicians sauntering the halls of the Venetian and gambling in its sparkling casino seemed blissfully unaffected by the criticism. One anti-aging doctor presented a lecture titled "The New Growth Hormone Replacement Therapy." Others coached physicians on how to stay within the law while prescribing HGH.

In the main ballroom, San Diego anti-aging luminary Rothenberg spoke before a packed crowd on what he referred to as "hormone myths." One myth, he insisted, was that adult growth hormone deficiency is only seen in people who had pituitary problems beginning in childhood. Then he asked the audience, can growth hormone cause cancer to grow? "Again, that is a myth," Rothenberg said.

In 2009, the American Association of Clinical Endocrinologists (AACE) released new guidelines for the proper diagnosis and treatment of growth hormone deficiency—a document that A4M embraced as affirmation of the organization's philosophies. In response to queries about the Olshansky and Perls dispute, A4M stated: "After ten years of controversy and stifling debate curtailing the uses of GH in the anti-aging clinical setting for patients with a diagnosed growth hormone deficiency, the 2009 guidelines update by AACE offers a significant validation of the safety and efficacy of adult GH replacement therapy." The AACE's guidelines, however, dismissed anti-aging medicine, stating in boldface type, "Growth hormone is no 'fountain of youth.'" And Vance, who coauthored the guidelines, confirmed the AACE's position. "AACE does not support the use of GH for anti-aging," she said.

Klatz and Goldman continued to attack their critics. In August 2009, they filed a defamation suit in New York Supreme Court against Wikimedia Foundation, Inc., the nonprofit organization that manages the online encyclopedia known as Wikipedia (www.wikipedia.org). Klatz and Goldman were unhappy with many of the statements in Wikipedia's description of A4M, including what they called in their lawsuit "false and defamatory information" about their medical credentials.

In the suit, Klatz and Goldman took issue with Wikipedia's description of a licensing dispute with the state of Illinois. As the Wikipedia page pointed out, Klatz and Goldman had received their M.D. degrees in 1998 from Central American Health Sciences University in Belize—degrees that were not recognized by Illinois licensing authorities. Klatz and Goldman were doctors of osteopathic medicine, which gave them the considerably less lauded D.O. title. In 2000, the Illinois Department of Professional Regulation fined the men $5,000 apiece and ordered them to stop using the "M.D." designation after their names in Illinois. Everywhere else, however, they continued to call themselves M.D.s. They used the title on their Web site and brochures, and both listed "M.D." first among their credentials on the cover of their 2005 book *121 Ways to Live 121 Years . . . and More!*

In response to an inquiry about the Illinois licensing matter, A4M stated: "This ten-year-old administrative dispute, due to a complaint to the Medical Board from a business competitor, is a dead issue. It has in effect been superseded by a Confidential Non-Disciplinary Order, issued February 28, 2006, which stated: 'Dr. Goldman/Dr. Klatz are licensed physicians and surgeons of osteopathic medicine in good standing in Illinois for over 20 years, which allows them to practice and carry out all the duties equivalent to what a medical doctor, an M.D., may do in Illinois. Dr. Goldman/Dr. Klatz have valid M.D. degrees from a recognized medical school, a school which is on the World Health Organization's list of approved and sanctioned medical schools. In fact, said medical school graduates are currently undergoing M.D. residency training in the USA and worldwide.'" Klatz and Goldman went on to point out that they "are licensed as M.D.s in a number of countries outside the United States."

They even threatened the author of this book and "all parties involved" with a suit for "scandalous statements about A4M, or its founders."

One would think that Tarsus's financing of A4M's conferences should have inspired Klatz and Goldman to tone down their sales tactics, but apparently it did not. Klatz and Goldman seemed to welcome anybody who was willing to buy a booth at the trade show. They said the exhibit hall was the only commercial element of the conference, but everything at the conference looked like it was somehow tied into selling something. At the 2008 event, most of the evening workshops were presented by exhibitors or by companies that had bought full sponsorships for upward of $25,000.

The companies served wine and hors d'oeuvres as they made not-so-subtle sales pitches for their products, some of which had no connection whatsoever to life extension. During one Friday night workshop, for example, a company called Hoya ConBio marketed a tattoo-removal machine. Will Kirby, a Beverly Hills, California, dermatologist featured on the TV show *Dr. 90210*, showed slides of some of the 31,000 tattoos he had erased with Hoya's machine.

Entrepreneurs who were lucky enough to strike deals with Klatz and Goldman scored prime real estate at the Las Vegas conference. One of the show's sponsors was a company called Arasys. The Hawaii-based outfit made machines that aimed electron beams at patients' skin and muscles, which purportedly prevented blood cells from clumping together. Founder Xanya Sofra-Weiss insisted that the contraptions—priced between $18,000 and $63,000 and displayed in a gargantuan booth in the center of the exhibit hall—could build muscle mass, erase wrinkles, and perform other miracles. All patients had to do was lounge in a cushy recliner and let the beams wash over them. The diminutive redhead paced her booth, watching volunteers as they lay under the Arasys Perfector. "Yeah, there's an improvement," Sofra-Weiss said into her headset microphone, commenting on one volunteer's skin quality.

Arasys received a funding commitment of up to $500,000 from CapRegen, a company partially founded by Klatz and Goldman. "We're basically part of A4M," Sofra-Weiss said proudly. "Dr. Klatz is a visionary. He opened up the world for us. He gave me the opportunity to profit and get to the next level." How she defined the "next level" wasn't quite evident. There were no studies of her technology published in respected medical journals. And the company's glossy sales brochures—handed out at the conference by model-thin women dressed in skintight blue and green dresses—were incomprehensible. Read one: "Ion Magnum revitalizes the joints how certain MENS (one over a millionth of an ampere) frequencies offer the required supply of protons necessary to spin the ATPase enzyme that synthesizes ATP (cellular energy)."

Each year the show expanded, its growth seemingly immune to economic dips. Even though the 2008 event was held on the cusp of the worst recession in 30 years, more than 6,000 doctors, pharmacists, and entrepreneurs paid $1,000 apiece to hear lectures on the latest anti-aging research and to troll the trade show filled with hormones, devices, and diets. They crowded into seminars on topics ranging from the weighty ("The Coming Pandemic of Liver Cancer") to the wacky ("The Newly Rediscovered Anti-Aging Properties of the Amazing Sunshine Vitamin D").

On the first full morning of the event, attendees filed into the main ballroom, clamoring to find seats in time for the starring act. At 8:30 a.m., Robert Goldman and Ronald Klatz took the stage to thunderous applause. "I'm amazed at how effective we've been in 16 years," Klatz said to the standing-room-only audience. Klatz, dressed in a black suit and red tie, ticked off the organization's most recent accomplishments, reading studiously from a stack of papers that he held above the podium. A4M had launched two new publications, the *Bulletin* and *Anti-Aging Pulse*, he reported. It had produced a video for doctors extolling the virtues of anti-aging medicine, which he encouraged them to play nonstop in their waiting rooms.

Klatz had just returned from Dubai, where he had advised the World Economic Forum on the challenges of dealing with an aging population. He boasted that A4M had landed on the radar screen of the highly regarded group, which attracted international leaders and topflight CEOs to its annual meeting in Davos, Switzerland. "This is the bluest of blue blood, the establishment. They're desperately looking for new ideas," Klatz said, excitement rising in his voice as he fired up his crowd of doctor disciples. "You can be recognized as part of the solution, part of the answer!" (Klatz's critic Olshansky, who was also a member of the World Economic Forum, claimed that Klatz made no substantive comments during the Dubai meeting, and said—incorrectly—that he was the only doctor in the group.)

When Goldman lectured at the A4M conference, he presented his vision of what aging should be like, flipping through a crazy collection of slides to drive home his message. There was a photo of perennially young TV host Dick Clark, and actress Sophia Loren posing on her 70th birthday wearing nothing but earrings. "This is a very very exciting time to be involved in medicine," Goldman said. One of his slides summed up the rules of anti-aging medicine: "Don't get sick. Don't get old," read the first two rules. The third was simply a picture of a skull and crossbones, with no words to explain. Goldman said the significance was clear: "Don't die," he said.

On the third morning of the conference, Leonard Horowitz took the stage and declared that the world needed an alternative to antibiotics and vaccines. Horowitz was an advocate of using silver hydrosols—tiny particles of silver mixed with water—to boost immunity. He cited no scientific proof that his idea was valid, and his first PowerPoint slide displayed a bizarre warning: "The FDA and EPA may consider silver hydrosols of regulatory concern. These agencies are currently considering regulating silver hydrosols as 'pesticides,' in support of drug industrialists and in violation of Federal Rico Organized Crime law, due to their competitive success as germ killers."

Horowitz began by suggesting that he had been blacklisted from speaking at mainstream medical meetings, largely because he accused the U.S. government of covering up evidence that HIV and other plagues had been engineered in biological weapons labs. And he published books and papers blaming vaccines for causing health problems ranging from autism to his own eczema. As he preached to the hushed crowd in increasingly urgent tones, Horowitz, a former dentist, charged the drug industry with genocide. He flipped to a slide showing a *Time* magazine cover of an autistic boy, accompanied by Horowitz's own angry commentary: "The 'aliens' doing this to our children in the name of 'public health' and medicine are capable of doing ANYTHING!" the slide read.

Horowitz then called for volunteers from the audience to form a prayer circle on the stage. He explained his theory that music at a certain frequency mixed with water could act as a universal healer. He passed among the volunteers a glass of water that he said was infused with a "nano-frequency" that made it "supercharged with love." He promised that such prayer sessions would free humanity from pathology. One woman dipped her finger in the cup and squealed. "You've just been zapped with love," Horowitz cried. "Have a wonderful day."

As Horowitz's prayer-filled diatribe drew to a close, Klatz made his way back to the stage for an impromptu editorial. He reminded the audience that A4M provided an unbiased forum for all thoughts related to disease and aging. Horowitz's ideas "may never be part of the mainstream," Klatz conceded. "But if we do not open our minds, we are so much poorer." The audience applauded. "I appreciate you for being so open and generous," Klatz continued. "This is a necessity for the future of health care."

CHAPTER 3

Too Tempting to Resist

In January 2000, Florida physician William Abelove of the Renaissance Longevity Center sent a letter to Fred Hassan, CEO of Pharmacia & Upjohn, one of five pharmaceutical companies that sold HGH. Abelove wrote that he was forming a strategic alliance that would include investment bankers, venture capitalists, and top marketing executives. His intention, he wrote, was to initiate "the most aggressive ethical campaign ever launched for the marketing of human growth hormone injections." Abelove invited Pharmacia to join the alliance. The group planned to use TV ads and "extensive public relations" to market HGH. Even though Pharmacia's product, Genotropin, was not FDA-approved to fight aging, Abelove's invitation—on letterhead bearing the name of his clinic, no less—made it obvious that he intended to prescribe it for that purpose. "We would like to arrange a meeting with you at the highest possible level at our headquarters in South Florida," wrote Abelove at the close of his letter.

Promoting HGH for anti-aging purposes was illegal—both for drug companies and for physicians—so Hassan should have thrown Abelove's letter in the trash. Instead, the CEO scribbled a note on top for his marketing staff to "follow up." Two of the company's executives hopped on a plane to Fort Lauderdale, Abelove said, and met him at a hotel. "They were very interested," Abelove recalled. "They invited me to be a consultant in their growth hormone program for adults. That started a chain of events." Abelove sent similar letters to four other HGH manufacturers, he said, but Pharmacia was the only one that responded.

With that single meeting, Pharmacia ventured into a risky but potentially profitable market. As a remedy for short children, HGH wasn't going to make anyone all that much money: The total market amounted to about $1 billion in sales a year. But once HGH was also approved to treat adult growth hormone deficiency, doctors could easily prescribe the hormone to just about any aging person who complained of being off his game. Physicians simply had to find a justification for their HGH prescriptions, so they could steer clear of the FDA or any other regulators who might be on the prowl for illegal off-label prescriptions.

But the companies themselves had to be a little more creative. It has always been illegal in the U.S. for pharmaceutical makers to engage in off-label marketing, so regulators were constantly looking for bad actors. Nevertheless, it would take years for them to recognize the rampant off-label use of HGH and to finally start pursuing those who promoted it.

After Abelove's meeting with Pharmacia, the company embraced him as its newest HGH consultant. Executives invited him to participate in the Kabi International Growth Study and

Kabi International Metabolic Study (KIGS/KIMS), a pair of research programs focused on children and adults taking Genotropin. They flew him to a meeting at a ritzy hotel in Monte Carlo, where they asked him to present his research on the use of growth hormone in adults, he said. "I didn't give an actual paper," Abelove recalled. "I talked about my experience with 100 adults I had treated with growth hormone." Pharmacia even sent the unassuming physician to Toronto for several days of media training, so he could appear on TV as a growth hormone expert, he said. And they sought his advice on HGH marketing strategies. During the first year of their partnership, Pharmacia paid Abelove $50,000 in consulting fees.

For any doctor struggling to stand out in the anti-aging mecca of south Florida, a Pharmacia partnership would be a golden opportunity. For Abelove, it seemed like the high point of a love affair with growth hormone that had started in the 1950s, when he was a trainee at Jefferson Medical College in Philadelphia. Back then, Abelove had helped treat a pregnant patient who had had a tumor on her pituitary gland and, as a result, too much growth hormone. She developed acromegaly, but much to Abelove's amazement, she was still able to deliver a healthy baby. He published a paper about the case in an endocrinology journal in 1954 and continued to read up on the hormone after he started his own internal medicine practice.

After HGH hit the market in the 1990s, Abelove started prescribing it to adults who had a combination of what he deemed to be low levels of growth hormone and incurable malaise. "These people had not responded to other forms of therapy—testosterone, thyroid, anti-depressants, God only knows what else," Abelove said. "And they got better. So I felt I was not doing them any harm." At the age of 70, he started taking growth hormone himself—a habit he would continue, on and off, for more than a decade.

Abelove didn't discuss the risks of off-label marketing with anyone at Pharmacia. "I don't think they brought it up. They were clearly interested in the adult market," he said. Indeed, in 1999, Pharmacia produced a brochure for patients titled *A Closer Look at Adult Growth Hormone Deficiency.* The colorful flyer, adorned with cartoons, said that adults with growth hormone deficiency "may feel tired" and "may experience an increase in body fat." It referred patients to a Web site (now defunct), www.growthhormoneinfo.com. "Pharmacia & Upjohn would like to help you learn more about staying healthy," the flyer stated. Nowhere did the company indicate that adult growth hormone deficiency is not a common problem— and most people with fatigue, body fat, and a general interest in staying healthy probably didn't have it. "Did I think it was off-label?" Abelove pondered. "Well it had to be off-label, because the FDA only approved [HGH] for adults who had a previous history of radiation or surgery on the pituitary and were growth hormone deficient. My patients did not meet that criterion."

Abelove pointed out that he was hardly a lone wolf in his pursuit of anti-aging medicines. "Over the years, at least a dozen physicians in south Florida contacted me, ostensibly because they wanted to take growth hormone themselves," said Abelove, whose quiet nature and noticeably unmuscular physique belied his obvious pride in his status as an HGH trailblazer. "I made available to them my protocols—how I prescribed the growth hormone, the dosage, how I followed [patients], the sources of the growth hormone. Just about every one of these guys went into the anti-aging business themselves."

It would take one daring marketing executive to bring to light the inappropriate promotion of human growth hormone. Peter Rost, a gregarious Swede with piercing blue eyes and a long résumé in medical marketing, had recently landed a $600,000-a-year job as vice president in charge of Pharmacia's endocrine care unit. He had no reason to suspect anything was amiss until a memo from a higher-up dated May 21, 2001, landed on his desk. Titled "Growth Hormone in Aging Patients," the memo declared in bold letters: "Pharmacia does not, may not and will not promote or encourage the usage of our products outside the approved labeling." Rost was puzzled. "It was unusual, this one-and-a-half-page memo," he said, because it seemed unnecessary to tell a seasoned pharmaceutical executive not to market a drug off-label. "It was like seeing a note on the refrigerator saying, 'We do not kill children, and we don't murder at all.'" Rost said. "It's natural. Why were they saying it? Something was not right."

Rost began to dig, and what he uncovered disgusted him. In 2000 and 2001, Pharmacia's U.S. sales of Genotropin totaled $184 million—and as much as 60 percent of adult sales appeared to be from off-label uses. About half of the drug's sales force was assigned to generating adult patients, according to internal sales charts. This seemed excessive, especially given that Rost's own calculations also showed that profit margins on the adult doses were actually negative. That is, Pharmacia lost money on each sale, because anti-aging doctors were prescribing smaller doses to adults than pediatric endocrinologists generally gave to children. "The incentives the sales reps received, compared to the revenues the drug brought in, didn't make it profitable," Rost said. Furthermore, he feared, if the company was caught promoting the drug off-label, its employees and customers could have faced up to five years in federal prison. "It was stupid," said Rost of the company's pursuit of the adult market, "and unprofitable."

Rost dug deeper and discovered other oddities. Abelove wasn't the only anti-aging doctor Pharmacia partnered with, Rost said. Pharmacia was paying hundreds of other doctors to collect data on patients for the KIGS/KIMS studies—$200 per patient enrolled, plus $200 for every year the patient stayed in the study. And the company was bankrolling an annual conference for more than 600 doctors in the Caribbean. But Rost wasn't entirely sure Pharmacia was doing anything with the KIGS/KIMS data. In fact, he had very strong opinions about this. He wondered if the doctors were researchers at all, or just recipients of cash rewards for diagnosing and treating adult growth hormone deficiency. That would constitute illegal kickbacks, Rost concluded. "I have documents from the study manager saying, 'This is not a study. It's just a database,'" Rost said. "Big difference. If it's not a study, then you can't call the people who input data 'investigators.' You can't pay them to go to the Caribbean. Suddenly all of that stuff becomes kickbacks—very illegal."

What Rost never doubted was that the partnerships were yielding new sales in the adult market. A slide created for a sales meeting showed that the company gained more than 100 new adult patients in January 2001 alone. Another slide suggested methods for generating even more sales. "Attempt to promote/distribute product through alternative channels (such as the Internet)," it read, "to focus on alternative indications (such as Healthy Aging)." Sales logs and attorney memos collected by Rost listed orders from more than 15 anti-aging clinics and pharmacies, including Renew Youth Centers in Atlanta, Georgia; Heartwise Fitness Institute in Whittier, California; and Hopewell Pharmacy in Hopewell, New Jersey.

Rost voiced his concerns to his supervisors, and in February 2002, they launched an internal investigation. Pharmacia promptly terminated all its contracts with anti-aging physicians. Just five months later, pharmaceutical giant Pfizer announced it would buy Pharmacia in a deal worth $58 billion. Rost continued to hound Pfizer's top executives about what he saw as the inappropriate marketing of HGH.

But Rost's own behavior would turn out to be his biggest handicap. In January 2003, the *New York Times* reported that Rost had filed a lawsuit against his former employer, Wyeth, alleging he had been demoted after uncovering evidence the company had cheated on its foreign taxes. (The dispute was later settled.) Then he started speaking out publicly for proposed legislation that would allow cheap drugs to be imported from Canada and other countries. Pharmaceutical companies despised that idea because they feared the plan would cut into their profits. As Rost became more and more of an industry gadfly, he found himself increasingly ostracized at Pfizer.

Figuring he had nothing to lose, Rost decided to blow the whistle on Pfizer. In June 2003, he filed a *qui tam* action against the drug giant in the U.S. District Court for the District of Massachusetts. In *qui tam* cases, individuals who believe they have evidence of corporate fraud can bring suits against companies on behalf of the United States. Rost's suit alleged that by marketing Genotropin off-label for children and adults, the company had violated federal and state statutes meant to shield Medicare and Medicaid from false claims. If Rost prevailed, he might earn enough to retire permanently: In the 14 years following a 1986 amendment to the False Claims Act, the U.S.

Justice Department recovered $1.5 billion in payments from companies that improperly billed government health plans. Whistle-blowers were awarded between 15 and 25 percent of those settlements.

But what Rost didn't know was that just two weeks earlier, Pfizer, in a letter the company sent to the FDA's Office of the Inspector General, had already confessed to distributing Genotropin to anti-aging doctors and pharmacists. Pfizer would later point to that confession as a justification for asking the government to throw out the case.

What Pfizer put Rost through next was like the corporate version of purgatory. The company slowly dismantled his 60-person department, moving everybody from Peapack, New Jersey, to Pfizer's New York City headquarters. "One by one my direct reports disappeared," Rost recalled. "Nobody called me. They just started to report to other people. They assigned two supervisors to me, and those people didn't return my phone calls." Eventually no one was left in the Peapack office except for Rost and his secretary, he said. Then, in 2004, men in hard hats showed up at the door. "They started knocking down the walls in the entire building around us," Rost said. "It was like something out of a movie."

In November 2005, the U.S. Attorney's Office in Boston declined to intervene in Rost's whistle-blower suit, greatly diminishing his chances of receiving either a massive payout or the glory of having exposed illicit corporate behavior. A month later, Pfizer fired him. But Rost refused to back down. He continued to fight the whistle-blower action on his own. And he filed a wrongful-termination suit against Pfizer.

Some of the documents unsealed in Rost's lawsuit indicated that Pfizer executives knew courting anti-aging doctors could get them into hot water. On February 7, 2000, the law firm Morgan, Lewis & Bockius sent one of Pharmacia's lawyers a six-page memo titled "Outline of Regulatory and Legal Implications of Possible Arrangements with Renaissance Longevity Center." The memo noted that in 1999, HGH maker Genentech had pled guilty to federal criminal charges of marketing growth hormone for five unapproved uses, including as a treatment for kidney disorders and burns. "Additionally, inducements were given by the company to physicians, which were found to be kickbacks," the memo warned. It went on to advise Pharmacia not to give physicians "cash payments or free goods as a result of conducting any research studies."

Nevertheless, Pharmacia continued to explore anti-aging opportunities. Just before its marketing executives flew to Florida to meet with Abelove in 2000, the doctor faxed them a letter laying out his hopes for the partnership. "I have written a book on longevity with a substantial focus on growth hormone being published in mid to late February," Abelove informed them. "It is possible that your products, with specific brand names, could be included in the book." In May of that year, Abelove landed the consulting agreement with Pharmacia.

The DOJ continued to investigate Pharmacia's marketing of Genotropin, even after stepping away from Rost's *qui tam*. And in April 2007, Rost scored a bittersweet victory. Pharmacia pled guilty to a single count of offering to pay a vendor to induce that vendor to recommend Pharmacia's products. Pfizer paid a fine of $19.7 million. At the same time, the company admitted that Pharmacia had promoted Genotropin for off-label uses such as anti-aging and paid a fine of $15 million. The company agreed to 36 months of federal monitoring. "It is important for the public to recognize that growth hormone has not been shown to be safe and effective for anti-aging, cosmetic or ath-letic uses, and it must not be promoted for such uses," said U.S. Attorney Michael J. Sullivan in a statement released by the DOJ. Sullivan went on to praise Pfizer for reporting the im-proper marketing activities in 2003.

In an online posting, Rost bitterly dismissed the settlements as "equivalent to a speeding ticket." He noted that Pfizer's profit the previous year had been $11 billion, so the $35 mil-lion in penalties amounted to nothing more than one day's profit for the pharma giant. In fact, as corporate hand-slaps go, it was pretty weak. In 2009, Pharmacia pled guilty to charges of marketing its pain drug Bextra off-label, and Pfizer paid the government $1.19 billion—the largest criminal fine ever. Whistle-blower John Kopchinski pocketed $51.5 million in that case. An earlier case against a different Pfizer subsidiary had resulted in a $430 million fine and earned a whistle-blower $26.6 million.

But because the government and Pfizer settled the Genotropin case independently of Rost's *qui tam*, the banished executive received nothing. Instead, his suit got tangled in an endless stream of motions and appeals. In November 2007, the Massachusetts district court dismissed the action, saying Rost had failed to provide enough details about the alleged fraud. Then a federal appeals court overturned the dismissal, and Rost filed an amended complaint, which included details of 200 al-legedly false claims filed in Indiana for the treatment of short children. In September 2008, a judge ruled that Rost could pro-ceed with the whistle-blower suit—but focusing only on off-label marketing of HGH for children. Rost's dream of making millions from exposing the illicit use of Genotropin in anti-aging clinics was dead.

The odds were against Rost from the beginning. Anti-aging was a cash business, so patients paid doctors and pharmacies directly, rarely filing claims to Medicare, Medicaid, or any other insurance plan. The few claims that were filed were coded as "adult growth hormone deficiency," a legitimate disease. Bottom line: No independent company was tracking prescriptions of Genotropin for anti-aging use. And that made it nearly impossible for Rost to try to prove his allegation that Pfizer was profiting from off-label promotions.

Pfizer's tame punishment by the DOJ did little to stem the flow of HGH into the anti-aging market. In 2008, Olshansky and Perls—by then clear of their legal battles with A4M and free once more to act as watchdogs for the anti-aging movement—estimated that $2 billion worth of growth hormone was being distributed yearly for anti-aging and sports use. "If you put 'anti-aging' and 'human growth hormone' into Google, you get 1,500,000 hits," Perls griped. "Sales of growth hormone are going up 20 percent a year. That's not because of short stature."

Because doctors were prohibited from prescribing HGH off-label, the hormone was in a legal class all by itself. Federal legislators worried about the increasing popularity of HGH and steroids in sports, and they feared that young athletes were risking their lives by taking the drugs. So they enacted two amendments to the Federal Food, Drug, and Cosmetic Act. The first, implemented in 1988, made it illegal to distribute steroids and HGH except when ordered by a physician specifically to treat a disease. The amendment also empowered the government to seize property from those who broke the law and to imprison them for more than a year. The second amendment, enacted in 1990, reclassified steroids as controlled substances.

HGH—which, contrary to common public perception, isn't a steroid—was left under the jurisdiction of the FDA. But it was criminalized in a way that instantly put the fledgling anti-aging industry on watch. Distributing HGH for any use other than what the FDA had authorized became a felony, punishable with a five-year prison sentence.

But it was unclear what exactly the FDA authorized. When the agency approved Eli Lilly's HGH drug Humatrope for adult use in 1996, the product's label specified that it should be used to treat patients who were growth hormone deficient because of surgery, radiation therapy, trauma, or diseases affecting the pituitary or hypothalamus. Over the next decade, another half-dozen HGH brands were approved for adult use, including Genotropin in November 1997. All the labels stated that the diagnosis of adult growth hormone deficiency "usually" required "an appropriate growth hormone stimulation test," a rather involved, four-hour process, during which patients must have a growth-hormone-releasing chemical infused intravenously and then have their blood tested every 30 minutes.

Some anti-aging doctors seemed to treat the word "usually" as permission to look beyond the guidelines. Instead, they adopted a much simpler blood test that measured IGF-1, which the body makes in response to growth hormone. The anti-aging industry established its own standards, embracing the idea that any patient with an IGF-1 level below 100 nanograms per milliliter of blood was a candidate for HGH. In his book *Grow Young with HGH*, Klatz recommended that patients strive to achieve IGF-1 levels similar to those of 30- to 35-year-olds, who typically scored as high as 492 on the test. But he and his followers didn't win any support from the FDA, the American Association of Clinical Endocrinologists, or the Endocrine Society, all of which published guidelines discouraging the widespread diagnosis of adult growth hormone deficiency based on IGF-1 results alone.

What's more, some doctors believed IGF-1 testing was notoriously unreliable. "Most of the IGF-1 assays are not sensitive, are not precise, and have a very poor reproducibility," said Cedars-Sinai endocrinologist Shlomo Melmed. Part of the problem, he explained, is that the body secretes growth hormone in a pulsatile fashion. "If you draw blood and measure growth hormone at the time of a pulse, you may have a very high level. If you draw at the time of a valley you'll have a very low level. So a single test may not tell you anything." Studies also showed that the quality of IGF-1 testing varied wildly depending on the type of assay used and the particular lab performing the test. "So Dr. X in Nevada who's running an anti-aging clinic measures a single IGF-1 level and says, 'Ah it's low, therefore I can give the patient growth hormone,'" Melmed said. "That is not a valid test."

Anti-aging doctors brushed off such criticism by stressing that they made their treatment decisions based largely on symptoms, not IGF-1 blood levels. Noting the diagnosis "adult growth hormone deficiency" in the charts of patients to whom they prescribed HGH and detailing symptoms that might be remotely related to a dearth of the magical hormone helped keep them off the radar screens of regulators.

In February 2006, San Diego's Ron Rothenberg moderated a conference for new anti-aging doctors at a seaside Holiday Inn in San Diego, which was sponsored by University Compounding

Pharmacy, a major supplier of HGH to anti-aging clinics. Rothenberg told the 166 attendees that they could diagnose HGH deficiencies based on a variety of symptoms—fatigue, increased body fat, and so on. Bounding enthusiastically across the stage, too antsy to stay behind the podium, he said, "You can explain in the charts that it's your clinical decision." He went on to say that physicians must properly document such diagnoses as adult growth hormone deficiency rather than as something HGH has not been approved to treat, such as chronic fatigue. He briefly addressed concerns about side effects, but suggested that any minor complaints reported by patients might not actually be caused by the drug.

Lawmakers struggled to gain traction against anti-aging physicians because so many of them used the diagnosis of adult growth hormone deficiency. But that didn't stop the FDA and others from trying to crack down on the anti-aging industry. The FDA's office of criminal investigations pursued 55 HGH cases in 2005—quadruple the number of cases it had explored in 2000. And it worked with the DEA and several other federal agencies to launch Operation Raw Deal, which was designed to dismantle suppliers of HGH and steroids. The operation yielded 124 arrests.

In 2006, the FBI's healthcare fraud unit in Connecticut started Operation Phony Pharm, aimed at people who were selling steroids and HGH over the Internet without legal prescriptions. Among those convicted was Alan Blair, who allegedly sold HGH from 2004 to 2007 via his Web site. His customers received HGH directly from a Chinese supplier, prosecutors said. Blair pled guilty, agreed to forfeit $260,000 of illegal proceeds, and in November 2008 was sentenced to two years of probation.

Anti-aging foes such as Perls and Olshansky urged federal lawmakers to make HGH a Schedule III controlled substance, which would require anyone who distributed it to register with the DEA. Changing HGH's classification would also stiffen the penalties for those caught prescribing it off-label. Bills in favor of that idea were introduced in both the Senate and the House in 2007, but neither made it out of committee before a change of administration shifted power and priorities in Washington.

On February 16, 2005, anti-aging doctor James Forsythe and his wife were sitting at the breakfast bar in their tony Reno, Nevada, home when they saw four black SUVs pulling up their steep driveway. They weren't expecting visitors, so Forsythe ran down the hall and opened the back door. He was met by 16 federal agents in stocking caps and flak jackets bearing the insignias "FDA" and "ICE," the initials of the Immigration and Customs Enforcement division of the U.S. Department of Homeland Security. "I looked at them and said, 'Is this a joke?'" recalled Forsythe, who was then 66 years old and practicing as an oncologist and anti-aging physician at the nearby Century Wellness Clinic. They held a gun to his chest, pushed him back into the house, forced him to kneel on the floor, and began to frisk him. "We have a search warrant for the illegal distribution of an unapproved drug through interstate commerce, for smuggling and money laundering," one of the agents told the doctor. When Forsythe's wife, Earlene, asked why her husband was being interrogated, an agent held a gun to her chest, too, and told her it was for the off-label prescribing of human growth hormone.

At first glance, Forsythe seemed a most unlikely criminal. A former army officer, Forsythe had served as a pathologist in Vietnam before moving to Reno to start an oncology practice in the mid-1970s. In 2001, he was searching for a way to ease into the twilight of his career when he happened upon A4M. "As you go into your retirement years, oncology is a very tough practice," said Forsythe, a soft-spoken man with a gravelly voice and a ready laugh. "You're dealing with terminally ill patients, families, all the complications that cancer patients endure. After a while, you've had enough. I liked the idea of holistic medicine, preventing disease, being able to enhance the quality of aging."

Forsythe only treated about 20 patients with HGH, and he never suspected he might be breaking the law. After all, he had learned at A4M conferences that prescribing growth hormone to old people wasn't any different than giving insulin to diabetics. Taking A4M's seminars earned him continuing medical education credits, which were accepted by his state's medical board. "I guess you can blame me," Forsythe said. "I had no concept I was doing anything illegal."

But the way Forsythe prescribed HGH should have been illegal. Instead of writing prescriptions for HGH, he stocked an Israeli-made version of the hormone in his office and sold it directly to patients. Lawyers who advised the anti-aging industry often debated whether the prohibition against "distributing" HGH protected anti-aging doctors who were merely "dispensing" it by writing prescriptions. But there was no gray area when it came to Forsythe: Once he started stocking HGH and selling it directly to patients, he became a de facto distributor.

Prosecutors often went after the little guys first, hoping to set a precedent that would discourage bigger players from acting illegally. Forsythe looked like the ideal candidate: a doctor selling HGH openly—and naively. "I was getting the drug from a pharmacy distribution center in Carson City, and they were licensed," Forsythe said. He had visited the company, which had been recommended to him by a patient, and had felt certain it was legitimate. Sure, some of the labeling was in Hebrew and Arabic, but it was a win-win arrangement for Forsythe, he figured. He could offer lower prices to his patients while at the same time increasing his profit margins.

Forsythe's legal troubles started in September 2004, when undercover FDA agent John Zelinsky showed up in an exam room at the Century Wellness Clinic, posing as a new patient. Zelinsky, who was in his mid-forties and had traveled to the clinic from Oakland, California, told Forsythe that he had recently been treated for a benign lung tumor. Ever since then, he had suffered from migraines, he was tired and depressed, and he had no tolerance for exercise. Zelinsky asked him about HGH, and Forsythe said that he ordered him to go to a lab and get an IGF-1 test. But rather than waiting for the results of the test, Forsythe sold him a vial of HGH on the spot, for $238, recounted Zelinsky in an affidavit supporting the search warrant. When Zelinsky came back for his second appointment, he still hadn't had the test, Forsythe said. Nevertheless, according to the affidavit, Forsythe sold Zelinsky a second vial of HGH. Forsythe said Zelinsky eventually got his IGF-1 levels tested. "It did show he was low," Forsythe said. "Of course, we're all low as we age."

Forsythe didn't see Zelinsky again until the day of the raid. While agents were holding the doctor and his wife at gunpoint at home, Zelinsky was at Forsythe's clinic, which was located in the back of a medical complex on a street lined with strip malls. Forsythe begged agents at his home to let him go to the office so he could explain the debacle to his patients. The agents searched his car for weapons and then let him go. By the time Forsythe got to his clinic, Zelinsky and his crew had already told patients they should find new doctors. 'Dr. Forsythe is engaged in criminal activity,' Forsythe said the agents told patients. Then the agents searched Forsythe's office, herded all his employees into one room, and called them out one by one to question them. The agents were brash and boorish, Forsythe said. Whenever the phone rang, one of them would pick it up and answer "Taco Bell."

Bonnie Brophy's husband was buying a vial of HGH for her at Forsythe's office when the agents burst through the door. They refused to give him the hormone. Brophy had been Forsythe's patient for 25 years. She had first started seeing him when she developed cancer in her right leg. The doctor cured her with chemo. Then, in 2001, she developed chronic fatigue syndrome and Lyme disease, making her sick and exhausted; "I was ready to cash in my chips," she said. Forsythe sold her HGH, which she injected regularly until the day of the raid. Brophy, who was in her mid-fifties at the time, said HGH changed her life. "I could get off the couch," Brophy said. "I could dig in the garden. My joints didn't hurt near as bad as they did before." Brophy was stunned by the revelation that prescribing HGH might make Forsythe a criminal. "It was scary. I stopped taking it."

In September 2006, Forsythe was indicted for importing HGH from Israel without FDA approval and for distributing it to treat something other than a recognized medical condition. He was fingerprinted, photographed, and held in a jail cell at the federal courthouse in Reno, until a judge released him on bond later that day. Forsythe's lawyer urged him to accept a misdemeanor at the minimum, and possibly a felony on his corporation. "Well, a felony on the corporation is a felony on me. My license would be taken away," Forsythe said. "It was unacceptable." So he fired his lawyer and instead hired Kevin Mirch, who had a reputation for taking on risky cases.

During the trial, which began a year later, Mirch systematically dismantled the government's case against Forsythe—and more importantly, the credibility of the agent chosen to lead it. In a motion to dismiss, he explained that the Israeli version of HGH that Forsythe was selling had been properly registered with the FDA, albeit under a different brand name than the one Zelinsky had seen on his prescription. Furthermore, Mirch said, Forsythe purchased it from Pharmacy International, a company licensed by the Nevada Board of Pharmacy. Therefore the doctor was neither importing it nor introducing it into interstate commerce, Mirch argued. Mirch's cross-examination of Zelinsky revealed that the agent had once worked at the FBI, where he had earned a reputation for being overly zealous, Forsythe said.

Perhaps the most damaging hit came when Mirch discovered that the government's evidence collection included HGH prescribed by Mark Gunderson, a Nevada physician with no affiliation to Forsythe. Someone had allegedly tried to scratch out Gunderson's name with a felt pen, but it was clearly visible when a light was shone on the ink markings. Zelinsky testified that he didn't know how a different doctor's HGH ended up in the chain of evidence, Forsythe said. "To me that was the breaking point of the trial," he said. "That's called tampering with evidence." Mirch skewered Zelinsky during the cross-examination, Forsythe said. "He didn't look good on the stand. The jurors were rolling their eyes."

Mirch felt so confident he had won the case that he didn't even bother presenting a defense. Halfway through the trial, the judge threw out the first count of the indictment, leaving only the charge of improper distribution. On day seven of the trial, November 1, 2007, the jury was ready to return its verdict. "I tried to read them as they came in the door, but I couldn't tell for sure," Forsythe recalled. The foreperson said, "Not guilty." Forsythe cried with relief. The allegations had cost him his hospital privileges, his malpractice insurance, and contracts with every major health plan that had been sending him new patients. Finally he could envision getting all that back, along with his reputation. "I was elated," he said.

Anti-aging critics said Forsythe's win proved how ill-equipped the FDA was to prosecute HGH cases. "The case fell apart," said Boston University's Perls. The professor had been working as a consultant to the DEA, reviewing medical records seized from anti-aging clinics and offering his opinion as to whether the drugs they prescribed were appropriate. Because HGH was under the purview of the FDA, Perls and his DEA contacts had no choice but to watch the Forsythe trial unfold from the sidelines. "It was the FDA that botched it," Perls said. "Forsythe came off as the kindly old doc who wanted to do all these wonderful things for patients. In front of the jury, he won them over. Growth hormone should be the jurisdiction of the DEA, not the FDA."

In April 2008, Mirch was disbarred in Nevada for filing what the state bar considered to be a frivolous case against another attorney. He would have to wait three years to petition the court for a reinstatement. But he retained his license in California, and he filed a case against the FDA on Forsythe's behalf. The suit alleged 11 violations on the part of the agency, ranging from assault and excessive force to slander and malicious prosecution. Forsythe hoped to win a monetary settlement, to help offset the millions he had lost in legal fees and unrealized patient revenues. But on January 25, 2010, a judge for the U.S. District Court for the Northern District of California dismissed the charges.

Doctors continued to prescribe HGH as the new fountain of youth, as would-be whistle-blower Rost struggled to bring attention to off-label promotion of the increasingly popular drug. In 2009, beaten down by his endless legal morass, his blue eyes framed by bags, Rost expressed some regret about how he had blown the whistle. If he had to do it again, he said, he would go straight to the authorities rather than discussing the issue with his supervisors. He was scraping together a meager living with some occasional writing and public speaking and by serving as an expert witness in pharmaceutical cases. He speculated that his whistle-blower suit would require at least a year more of discovery before it could progress any further. His employment case was inching along, too, but he was bracing himself for what might happen if he won. "Pfizer will appeal," he predicted. "They're doing everything they can to drag things out."

Pharmacia didn't renew Abelove's consulting contract, and in 2001 the company sued him, claiming he didn't pay for all the Genotropin he received. Abelove settled the suit for $95,520, which he paid off in monthly installments of $750. He never heard from Pharmacia or Pfizer again. He abandoned his book and his plans to launch Renaissance Longevity Center, but he continued to practice anti-aging medicine out of a small clinic in Weston, Florida. And he remained a fan of Genotropin. "It's the best product in the field," he said. He credited his own use of the hormone with giving him the energy to see 100 patients a week, even at the age of 81. "I don't have an associate. I'm in practice by myself," he said. "It's nice to be productive when you're in your eighties and you know you can help people."

Forsythe never lost his faith in HGH either. He injected the hormone for six years, stopping only after the federal investigation began. After he won the case, he started back up again. "I'm 70 years old. I have a very busy practice," he said. "I work seven days a week. I still play tennis three days a week. All my lipid profiles improved. I feel my exercise tolerance is better. It affects my libido. My cognitive function is as sharp as ever."

With the nightmare of his arrest behind him, Forsythe gingerly reenacted the raid that had disrupted his breakfast and opened his eyes to the perils of anti-aging medicine. He retraced his steps, walking from his kitchen, down the hall, past his home gym and infrared sauna, to the back door. He still wondered who had ratted him out to the FDA. Maybe it was a disgruntled employee who had worked in his billing department, he said, or perhaps someone was trying to get back at his wife, who had acquired quite a few political enemies while working as the chairwoman of Nevada's Republican Party. The shock of confronting a sea of federal agents was still fresh in his memory, but Forsythe could laugh about it then. He had regained privileges at two of the three hospitals where he had been practicing, and he had won back most of his insurance contracts. He was still prescribing HGH, though he was no longer selling it at his clinic. "I just prescribe it and let them get it at a pharmacy," he said. "I want to be squeaky clean."

Forsythe's victory over the Feds made him a deity in A4M circles. At the December 2008 conference in Las Vegas, Forsythe and Mirch led a full-day seminar on the ramifications of their not-guilty verdict. They enraptured the crowd with tales of federal agents searching the Forsythes' house for seven hours and escorting them to the shower and toilet to make sure they wouldn't escape. "I thought I was in Russia with the KGB, or in Nazi Germany," said Forsythe, gripping the sides of the podium as he stammered through the tale. An audience member gasped in amazement and whispered under his breath, "Scumbags."

Mirch told the crowd the lesson they should take away was clear: "You are not regulated by the FDA," he bellowed. "You guys get to practice any way you want." Mirch's final Power-Point slide read simply: "James W. Forsythe, M.D., is a hero."

CHAPTER 4

Homemade Sex Hormones

If anti-aging physicians had focused only on HGH, the industry would have gone the way of naturopathic medicine or chiropractic, becoming little more than a niche specialty and mostly sought out by he-men unafraid to chase down their youth with an unproven therapy. So anti-aging doctors began reaching out to the largest and most decisive segment of the healthcare-buying public—aging women. The strategy: to persuade them that hormones made from yams and soybeans were a much better cure for hot flashes and other menopausal symptoms than the "synthetic" hormones made by big pharma. For much of the previous half century, the reigning menopause remedy had been Wyeth's Premarin, which was derived from hormones in the urine of pregnant mares. Klatz, Goldman, and a few key allies began promoting the idea that pharmaceutical hormones were dangerous. Instead they suggested, all women should have anti-aging doctors design tailored doses of "natural" hormones, which were identical to what their bodies had made during their younger years.

The notion that yams were somehow closer to humans than horses seemed ludicrous. But the anti-aging industry's propensity to persuade—coupled with their extraordinarily good timing—made for marketing magic. Anti-aging doctors promised patients they could replace waning hormones with mixtures of plant-derived estrogen and progesterone, which would not only turn off the menopausal sweat spigot but also reset the female body back to its younger self. Nearly 40 million female baby boomers were staring menopause in the face. And just as they had taken on every other challenge of their generation, they intended to fight it on their own terms. Natural hormones that were designed to fit perfectly into their bodies held so much more appeal than the one-size-fits-all Premarin pills their mothers had taken. Sex became a powerful selling point, too: Use natural remedies to restore your hormones to the levels they were in your twenties, and you'll enjoy sex as much as you did before you became a mortgage-paying soccer mom. Or so the physicians said.

Jonathan Wright, a doctor at the Tahoma Clinic in Renton, Washington, was the granddaddy of the alternative-hormone movement. Armed with a Harvard degree and an M.D. from the University of Michigan, Wright began practicing family medicine in the 1970s. But he was bothered by his inability to cure common ailments with drugs, so he started studying herbs and nutrition, always striving to combine alternative therapies with what he believed was the best of traditional medicine. Whenever a woman came in complaining of hot flashes, Wright did the only thing he knew how to do: He scribbled out a prescription for Premarin. One day in 1982, a patient read his prescription pad upside down as he was filling it out. "She looked at me and said, 'Do I look like a horse?'" Wright recalled. "'I want hormones that are identical to the ones that were in my body when I was in my twenties and thirties.'" For Wright, it was a revelation. "'Damn,'" he muttered to himself, 'why didn't I think of that?'"

Working with a handful of local pharmacists, Wright developed "triest," a cream containing the three types of estrogen that the female body makes naturally: estradiol, estriol, and estrone. He performed several tests on his patients, including saliva tests that required them to spit into tubes a few times a day, and he sent the samples out to labs. He claimed the labs could study the samples to pinpoint hormone deficiencies. Then he would ask pharmacists to make up drug mixtures designed to replace the hormones back to levels typically seen in young women.

At about the same time, a doctor in northern California named John Lee was prescribing plant-based progesterone cream and reporting that his menopausal patients loved it. So Wright added progesterone to his concoctions. Eventually he started throwing in other hormones, such as thyroid and testosterone—provided a patient's saliva test revealed she needed the boost. He called his mixtures "bio-identical" because they had the same structure as endogenous human hormones.

Wright was convinced that his hormones were better than anything the big pharmaceutical companies could offer. The only reason those companies weren't selling natural hormones, he told patients, was that they couldn't patent natural substances, so they couldn't make any money from them. "Patent medicine companies have done a marvelous job of blurring the lines," said Wright, who punctuated his speech with loud crescendos to show his obvious contempt for the drug industry. "They call it estrogen even if it's never been found in the human body," he said, "or in fact if it's never been found on planet EARTH before."

On May 6, 1992, 14 armed FDA agents kicked in the doors of Wright's clinic. They seized bottles of vitamins and herbs, as well as the office's electrodermal testing machines, which, Wright said, "are very useful for measuring body energy flows." Undercover agents who had been snooping around Wright's office for months found contaminated, moldy magnesium supplements in the clinic's dumpster, and they raised questions about the injectable B vitamins that Wright was importing from Germany. But the government had very little authority over how natural remedies were marketed, so the agents struggled to prove that Wright was doing something illegal. Three years and two grand juries later, a U.S. prosecutor failed to win an indictment against Wright. The government dropped the investigation.

Free from government oversight, Wright began to ride the anti-aging wave. He traveled around the country, teaching other anti-aging doctors to abandon "extraterrestrial estrogens" in favor of hormones made from plants. "Copy nature," Wright said, repeating a mantra he passed along to his pupils. "Don't use molecules that have never been found in nature. It is true that Premarin is found in nature, but it's found in horses, and the molecular size and shape is entirely different. CO-PY NA-TURE."

One of Wright's disciples and A4M's most effective salespeople was former emergency room doctor Pamela Smith. She discovered anti-aging medicine in 1993, when she suddenly came down with a terrible case of insomnia. The sleeplessness was more than a mere irritation to the 39-year-old hard-charging physician, who had been enjoying a career at the busy Detroit Medical Center. It was the kiss of death in a workplace where doctors were expected to save lives during the wee hours and to grab shut-eye at odd times so they'd be refreshed for the next shift. A desperate Smith consulted 11 doctors. They all told her to take a sleeping pill and get over it. Then one of her colleagues invited her to attend one of A4M's first conferences. During the second seminar, Smith learned that women often run low on progesterone and that the deficiency can cause insomnia.

When Smith returned home, she searched for a doctor who would give her a saliva test, and she was stunned to discover she had no progesterone at all. So she rushed to a pharmacy on the end of the block where she had grown up and asked the pharmacist to cook up capsules of natural progesterone, extracted from yams. The daily dosage was exactly what Smith needed, she believed, to replace what age had taken away. "In two days," Smith said, "I slept like a baby."

Smith opened a part-time practice to help women deal with the scourges of menopause: hot flashes, night sweats, insomnia, lack of sex drive. She told patients they could erase their symptoms by using bio-identical creams and capsules. She lured women to her practice by describing this new brand of menopause therapy during evening seminars in pharmacies and conference centers. Demand for her expertise grew so quickly that in 1999, Smith left her 22-year emergency room (ER) career behind and opened 27 anti-aging practices from Michigan and Illinois to Texas and Florida.

"Skin feeling crawly? . . . Can't find the keys?" Smith asked a crowd of 50 women, who gathered at the Scottish Rite Center in San Diego to hear her spiel. It's not just about hot flashes and cold libidos, Smith said. Dizzy spells, incontinence, indigestion, even back pain—they're all related to hormone imbalances, she claimed. Smith, a short woman with a sometimes-droll speaking style, was dwarfed by the huge podium on the stage.

But she enraptured the crowd with her tantalizing message: Hormones can be measured in spit and then replaced so that a woman feels as good as she did before menopause. They are natural, she said, and so much safer than Premarin. Smith would soon be called upon to preach to patients all over the country about the miracle of sweatless, sleep-filled, sexed-up nights. She spoke nearly every day, logging 250,000 miles a year on Northwest Airlines.

Smith's act was simply an updated version of a pro-hormone movement that the pharmaceutical industry had launched 50 years earlier. The notion that menopause is a disease that can be treated with drugs started with Premarin, which made its U.S. debut in 1942. Invented by Canadian company Ayerst, McKenna and Harrison, Premarin was pitched as a more potent, less toxic estrogen than the nausea-inducing and sometimes expensive hormones that had dominated the market until then.

Physicians hailed Premarin as a "natural" wonder, pristine in its origin, and so much closer to human than its chemical predecessors. Suddenly replacement hormones became elixirs that could do more than just free women from hot flashes. They could be taken in convenient pills every day for life, to prevent heart disease, perhaps, and osteoporosis—a permanent cure, in essence, for growing old. Wyeth, which bought Ayerst in 1943, began running ads in medical journals in the mid-1960s, depicting a stylishly dressed, wrinkle-free older woman with perfectly coiffed gray hair, chatting in a theater with two distinguished gentlemen. "Help keep her this way," the suggestive ads for Premarin read, adding that the drug was "specifically designed for estrogen replacement in the menopause . . . and later years."

Then, in 1966, New York gynecologist Robert Wilson published the book *Feminine Forever*, a 200-page love letter to pharmaceutical estrogen. Wilson rhapsodized about the hormone's magical power to prevent women's breasts and genitals from shriveling up. He promised readers it would reawaken long-dormant sexual desires, turning them back into tempting vixens and preventing their husbands from seeking out younger, perkier mates. "Women should not have to live as sexual neuters for half their lives," Wilson wrote. Estrogen from pregnant mares, he claimed, was the perfect therapy for all women, "to counteract the chemical castration that befalls her during her middle years."

The number of estrogen prescriptions skyrocketed from 15.5 million in 1966 to 28 million in 1975—70 percent of which were written for Premarin. Sales stalled briefly in the late 1970s after studies suggested that equine estrogens increased a woman's risk of uterine cancer. But doctors discovered they could protect the uterus by prescribing Premarin with Provera, which had been introduced by the Upjohn Company in 1959 to prevent miscarriages and treat irregular uterine bleeding. Provera was dubbed a "progestin," because it was a chemical copy of natural progesterone that was altered so patients could take it by mouth. Wyeth-Ayerst put the two hormones together in a convenient one-pill dose, which it introduced as Prempro in 1995. Sales for the Premarin/Prempro franchise jumped from under $200 million per year in the 1970s to nearly $2 billion in 2000.

Then in 2002, a single study sent shock waves through the field of women's health—and gave the anti-aging industry an unprecedented shove into the medical mainstream. A National Institutes of Health (NIH) trial called the Women's Health Initiative (WHI) discovered an increased risk of breast cancer in postmenopausal women who were taking Prempro compared to those taking a placebo. The danger was serious enough for the NIH to halt that arm of the trial three years earlier than planned. Investigators also found a 22 percent increase in heart disease and a 41 percent higher risk of stroke. Women on the combination therapy faced double the danger of suffering deep vein thrombosis and pulmonary embolism. Two years later, the Premarin-only arm was stopped, too, because even the solo hormone seemed to boost the risk of stroke and blood clots. Labels were slapped on Premarin and Prempro warning women of the perils and imploring them not to take hormones to prevent heart disease, heart attacks, strokes, or dementia. It was a stunning about-face from the *Feminine Forever* days, when hormone therapy was held up as the magical cure for the ravages of old age. Millions of women quit the hormones cold turkey: Pharmacies reported a 33 percent decline in Premarin prescriptions and a 70 percent drop in Prempro prescriptions.

For the boosters of bio-identicals, the panic spelled opportunity. Anti-aging doctors bad-mouthed Wyeth to patients, persuading millions of them that big pharma's synthetic hormones caused cancer because NATURE didn't intend for people to swallow equine estrogens. They calmed legions of terrified women by explaining that Prempro was bad because it contained both horse pee and proges-TIN, which is a fake and therefore dangerous version of nature's proges-TERONE, annunciating key syllables, as Wright did, to emphasize the difference.

Hormone creams made from yams and soybeans were an easy sell in a society that had grown obsessed with everything organic. In the early 2000s, healthy was hot. Americans flocked to natural grocery chains like Whole Foods Market, which was opening a dozen new stores a year and had seen its revenues double in five years, to $2.7 billion. Health insurers rarely reimbursed bio-identical brews. But the economy was booming, so it didn't seem unreasonable to ask patients to pay out of pocket, sometimes hundreds of dollars a month, for holistic hormones.

At the same time, mom-and-pop pharmacies were struggling to stay afloat as health insurers slashed reimbursement rates on expensive prescription drugs. For these entrepreneurs, the appeal of anti-aging medicine was undeniable: They could go into a back room, mix up hormones according to a doctor's instructions, and sell them straight to patients, cutting out the insurance middlemen. These pharmacists, known as "compounders," didn't answer to the FDA, so they didn't have to test their customized prescriptions for safety or efficacy.

Membership in the Professional Compounding Centers of America (PCCA), a trade group for independent pharmacies, started increasing at double-digit rates. A second trade group, the International Academy of Compounding Pharmacists (IACP), also ballooned. The FDA estimated that by 2003, more than 30 million prescriptions for compounded drugs were being written every year, with hormones among the three most popular products.

Yet the party line—that bio-identical hormones were natural and that drug companies didn't sell them because they couldn't patent them—was not the whole story. The truth is that big pharma was making plenty of its own plant-derived hormones, which were fully tested for safety and efficacy and approved by the FDA. Bayer introduced an estradiol patch called Climara in 1994, and rival Novartis had its own patch called Vivelle-Dot. There was also Estrasorb lotion from Esprit Pharma and EstroGel from Ascend Therapeutics. In 1998, Solvay Pharmaceuticals won FDA approval to market Prometrium, a capsule containing progesterone derived from yams. All these products were molecularly identical to what the human body made itself, and most of them came in a variety of doses, so doctors could adjust them according to the needs of each patient. Drug companies patented them based not on their natural building blocks but rather on how the end products were formulated and packaged into patches or gels. They just didn't call them "bio-identical."

The notion that compounded hormones were somehow different—somehow safer—than "synthetic" drug-company versions was an invention of the anti-aging marketing machine. It's as if the industry's leading players were creating a mirage of the friendly neighborhood pharmacist mashing up yams and soybeans and painstakingly mixing them into harmless lotions. The truth was that bio-identical estrogen and progesterone were chemical compounds, made from the very same raw materials that drug companies used to make their hormone drugs. The end products were nothing more than manufactured medicines, regardless of whether they were Prometrium and Vivelle-Dot made by chemists in pharmaceutical labs or bio-identical lotions made in the back rooms of pharmacies.

But the FDA could not impose the same marketing restrictions on the anti-aging industry that it could on drugmakers, so hype prevailed. Wright's Web site bragged that his Tahoma anti-aging clinic prescribed "hormones 'approved' by nature," which had benefited women with "osteoporosis, heart disease, and other problems." It went on to state, "Bio-identical hormone therapy is far and away less risky than the use of horse urine and progestins, which women should surely avoid." Pharmacists all over the country handed out bio-identicals without any printed warnings about side effects or instructions for how to use them.

By contrast, the Web sites for Vivelle-Dot, Prometrium, and all the other FDA-approved versions of bio-identicals prominently displayed dire warnings that the hormones raised the risk of heart attacks, strokes, breast cancer, blood clots, and dementia. "Do not use estrogens with or without progestins to prevent heart disease, heart attacks, or strokes," they went on to implore. The language was not much different from what Wyeth had to add to all its marketing material for Premarin and Prempro.

Compounding pharmacists knew that the hormones they were selling could be dangerous if not handled properly in their labs. Their own trade groups went to great lengths to warn them that if they mishandled hormones, they could get cancer. A 2002 issue of the trade newsletter the *Pharmacists' Link*, published by the International Academy of Compounding Pharmacists, reported that the Occupational Safety and Health Administration (OSHA) of the U.S. Department of Labor had increased its scrutiny of pharmacies. In response, IACP posted a detailed set of instructions on its Web site, referring to estriol, estradiol, estrone, and progesterone as hazardous chemicals that "are harmful if swallowed, inhaled or absorbed through the skin." The notice went on to state that hormones "can have chronic chemical effects on the body, including altering genetic material, causing cancer and heritable genetic damage," and it demanded that pharmacists cover their entire bodies—beards and eyes included—when working with the hormones. Yet when these same pharmacists handed finished hormone creams to patients, they faced no requirements to warn of any risks.

Margaret Polaneczky, an ob-gyn at Weill Cornell Medical College in New York, found that confusion was rampant among patients who demanded "natural" bio-identical hormones. So Polaneczky told them to imagine a chemical manufacturer's warehouse with two lines coming out of it. "One shows hormones going to Joe Blow Compounding Pharmacy, and he tells you they're safe," she said. "The other shows the same hormones going to the companies making drugs like Climara, and they put huge boxed warnings on them that scare the hell out of you."

Polaneczky didn't oppose compounded bio-identicals. On the contrary, she often prescribed them, and she used a specially tailored lotion of progesterone and estrogen to ease her own hot flashes. But she had ultrasound examinations regularly to check that her uterus was cancer-free—a precaution she urged all her patients to follow. Polaneczky got so tired of correcting misconceptions spread by the anti-aging industry that in 2004 she started "The Blog That Ate Manhattan" and used it as a forum to spout off on the bio-identical brouhaha. "Estrogen is estrogen," she wrote in one posting, "whether it comes from plants, mares' urine or the moon."

Of all the female hormones anti-aging doctors prescribed, estriol took on a special significance. Mainstream gynecologists called estriol the "weak" estrogen because it was 80 times less potent than estradiol. It was not contained in any FDA-approved drugs. Nevertheless, the anti-aging industry painted estriol as a menopause multitasking phenomenon, capable of doing everything from eliminating hot flashes to lubricating the vaginas of women who complained of being too dry down there to enjoy sex. Doctors told patients that estriol would shield them from cancer and Alzheimer's disease, too. "It's a very protective estrogen," Wright claimed. "When women are pregnant, they have MORE DARNED ESTRIOL—about a thousand times as much as when they're not pregnant. If that were dangerous we'd have a whole lot of damaged babies and a whole lot of sick women."

Yet science suggested estriol was neither the wonder drug nor the safe harbor that proponents like Wright claimed it was. To feed his estriol enthusiasm, Wright often pointed to a 35-year study that he said showed the hormone's significant role in protecting women against breast cancer. The reality is that the study looked at naturally occurring levels of estriol and other hormones in pregnant women only, and the researchers cautioned that their observations would need to be confirmed before anyone used estriol as a therapeutic tool. Estriol fans also quoted studies done in the 1960s and '70s by Henry Lemon at the University of Nebraska. But his most compelling evidence of breast protection came from studies of cell cultures and rats—subjects that are often poor predictors of what happens in actual humans. And in 1980, he published a report describing his own experience giving estriol to 24 women with breast cancer. Six of them saw their tumors grow. Two developed endometrial hyperplasia—a precancerous condition of the uterus. In one study of Dutch women who had undergone hysterectomies, vaginal estriol stimulated the abnormal growth of uterine cells.

Even though estriol was sold overseas in some menopause drugs, pharmaceutical companies never found much use for it in the United States. Anti-aging doctors, repeating their favorite refrain, said that was because drugmakers couldn't patent estriol. But the wealth of patented estradiol products proved otherwise. What is more likely, serious scientists surmise, is that estriol is so weak that it would be impossible to prove its worthiness in FDA-quality clinical trials without giving it in potentially dangerous doses. Even the estriol products sold overseas were rarely promoted as entirely risk-free. The label for Hormonin, a three-hormone drug containing estriol and sold in Europe, listed a number of cancer warnings and 15 side effects. It didn't promise that estriol would protect women from the adverse effects of the other estrogens, nor did it suggest that long-term use was smart.

The claims anti-aging doctors made about progesterone were equally suspect. Unlike the synthetic progestins, they said, natural progesterone acted as a barrier against heart disease and atherosclerosis, and it raised high-density lipoprotein (HDL), otherwise known as "good" cholesterol. They told patients that progesterone cream would protect them from the carcinogenic effects of estrogen. But there was no definitive proof any of that was true. The Postmenopausal Estrogen/Progestin Interventions (PEPI) trial—a study of 875 women sponsored by the NIH's National Heart, Lung, and Blood Institute (NHLBI) in the 1990s—found that all combinations of Premarin and progesterone raised HDL, regardless of whether the progesterone was an "-erone" or a "-tin." An NHLBI director cautioned, however, that more research would be needed to determine whether raising HDL would ultimately lower a woman's chances of developing heart disease. A 2005 meta-analysis of ten studies found no heart-protective benefit for any hormone therapy.

More disturbingly, a 2000 study by a team of Australian researchers found that progesterone cream provided no measurable protection for the uterus lining. Five years later, the lead investigator on that study, Barry Wren, examined eight trials of progesterone cream. He found little evidence that the hormone had been adequately absorbed or that it provided much relief for hot flashes, depression, low libido, or other classic signs of menopause. "The claims for transdermal progesterone creams and the hypothesis on which they are based have been founded on anecdotal information rather than on sound scientific research," Wren concluded in a paper published in the *Medical Journal of Australia.*

Progesterone promoters said the hormone protected women from breast cancer, but that was open to question. A French study of nearly 100,000 women suggested that breast cancer risk might be lower in women taking progesterone than in those on progestin. But it was an "observational" study, meaning it didn't involve a placebo arm. So the results were not as reliable as they would have been in a "randomized-controlled" trial (the preferred trial form) comparing progesterones, progestins, and placebos. And it's possible that the women who chose to use progesterone were different in other ways from those who picked progestins, and that may have affected their outcomes. The French investigators conceded upon releasing their findings in a 2008 edition of the journal *Breast Cancer Research Treatment* that "more evidence is required before these results can be translated into firm clinical recommendations for the management of menopausal symptoms."

Even the hormones that women's bodies make naturally can be dangerous. In 2002, University of North Carolina scientists published research in the journal *Cancer Epidemiology, Biomarkers and Prevention* showing that pregnant women with naturally high levels of all three estrogens combined relative to progesterone during pregnancy faced an increased risk of breast cancer. And there is compelling evidence that high endogenous levels of all of the sex hormones—estrogen, progesterone, testosterone, and others—are associated with breast cancer. As part of a research endeavor known as the Nurses' Health Study, scientists at Harvard examined blood samples from more than 1,000 nurses who were not taking any pharmaceutical hormones. They discovered that the nurses with the highest levels of naturally occurring hormones were the most likely to develop breast cancer.

Then there was the quality problem with compounded hormones. Because the FDA had little control over compounding, pharmacists didn't have to follow the same strict manufacturing standards for sterility, potency, and consistency that drugmakers did. Compounders were regulated by state pharmacy boards, which didn't have enough manpower to micromanage every little corner pharmacy. The result was a wide variation in quality, with no guarantee that patients were actually getting what their doctors were prescribing.

Ob-gyn Wulf Utian was horrified as he watched the bio-identical craze take hold. Utian, who began his career in his native South Africa, started the North American Menopause Society (NAMS) in 1989, with twin goals of educating women about menopause and fostering research into new remedies. The notion that hormones can be measured and then replenished to youthful levels was fundamentally flawed, he said. Hormone levels fluctuate moment to moment, day to day. Any attempt to measure them—by testing saliva samples collected several times during a single day, for example—yields nothing more than a snapshot in time. "If you want to match ideal levels, you'd need an IV pumping out hormones that's attached to a computer. There's no way to match it," he griped. Like most conservative doctors, Utian suggested that women use the lowest possible dose of whichever FDA-approved hormone

relieved their symptoms and then get off the drugs as soon as
they didn't need them anymore. It was safer, Utian said, than
constantly measuring their hormone levels and tweaking their
regimen of untested tinctures in a desperate attempt to chase
down their youth.

Utian's outspoken nature didn't win him many friends on
either side of the aisle. He was blasted for being an estrogen
critic when he voiced concerns about the rapidly growing use
of drugs like Premarin. Then he was labeled a big pharma hack
when he questioned the negative results found in the Women's
Health Initiative. In 2008, the compounding pharmacists skewered Utian on a Web site called CompoundingFacts.org
(www.compoundingfacts.org), put together by the IACP. NAMS
received funding from Wyeth and other pharmaceutical companies that made hormone products—a type of financial rela-
tionship that is hardly uncommon in the not-for-profit world.
But the pharmacists contended that Utian's viewpoints were
tainted by the payouts, which they said included a $200,000
Wyeth-endowed lectureship fund that was named after him.

Utian likened the marketing of compounded hormones to
that of a baker selling her own version of Oreo cookies but
telling customers they didn't cause obesity or cavities. "These
pharmacists are making mixtures that are not standardized or
supervised, throwing in extra stuff that's not approved by the
FDA, and making claims that are outrageous," Utian said.

Even some supporters of natural medicine were mystified
by how successful the anti-aging industry was at persuading
women that bio-identical hormones were safe. "Bio-identical
hormones are not from natural sources," said Adriane Fugh-
Berman, an associate professor of complementary and alternative medicine at Georgetown University who practiced

alternative medicine early in her career. "And you could argue that because Premarin is from pregnant horses, that's what's really natural."

Fugh-Berman was hardly an ally of the drug industry. She once chaired the National Women's Health Network, one of a handful of advocacy groups that refused to take donations from big pharma. She urged the FDA to reject Wyeth's attempts to get Premarin approved for preventing heart disease in the early 1990s. She directed PharmedOut.org, a project that exposed untoward marketing practices of major pharmaceutical companies.

But when anti-aging doctors and pharmacies started promoting bio-identical hormone therapy en masse, Fugh-Berman found herself siding with her big pharma foes. She wasn't concerned just with safety issues. She knew from her own experience as a doctor that there was no such thing as an optimal hormone level for easing the path through menopause. "There will be women with estrogen levels of zero who aren't having hot flashes, and there will be others that have hormone levels close to premenopausal women who are having terrible hot flashes," Fugh-Berman said. "If hormone levels are not directly connected to symptoms, why are they following hormone levels at all? Is it just to make more money, or is it to add a metric gloss to the whole endeavor? It's pseudoscientific."

On July 22, 2004, Fugh-Berman was invited to be a dissenting voice on bio-identicals at a congressional hearing. She had barely taken her seat when she realized she was in hostile company. Leading the hearing was U.S. Representative Dan Burton (R-IN), who began by expressing his disdain for "synthetic" hormones such as those studied in the recently halted Women's Health Initiative. "Barbara, my wife, was taking synthetic hormones when she contracted the breast cancer that eventually, at least in part, took her life, and I firmly believe that her overall health and quality of life deteriorated because she was taking those doctor-prescribed hormones," he sniffed during the hearing. He went on to parrot the unscientific claims about bio-identicals that so many anti-aging doctors were using to recruit patients. "Because these biologically identical hormones are the same chemical structure as the hormones created in the body," Burton said, "the body does not have the same harmful reactions as it does when the synthetic hormones are administered."

The testimony began with the NIH's Barbara Alving, who summarized the results of the Women's Health Initiative. Burton demanded to know who sponsored the study. Alving replied that one of the principal investigators had received funding from Wyeth. "OK, that's all I wanted to know," Burton snapped. "Pharmaceutical company. That's all I wanted to know." Then, inexplicably, Burton went on a rant about mercury in vaccines. "My grandson got autism after getting nine shots in one day, seven of which contained mercury," he said. "And now we're finding out that the synthetic estrogen caused problems probably more than it helped." Burton continued to pound Alving, asking her why Premarin and Prempro were still on the market. "It's the same reason that they haven't taken mercury out of vaccines," he surmised. "Mercury is one of the most toxic substances on the face of the earth." (Drug companies were no longer putting mercury in most vaccines. The chemical's link to autism has never been definitively proven.)

Fugh-Berman took the floor and began to lay out all the counterarguments on bio-identicals. Just as she started to explain the link between estriol and cancer, Burton cut her off and asked her to summarize the rest of her presentation so he could be sure to get to the other panelists. Then Burton asked whether Fugh-Berman or her advocacy group received funding from pharmaceutical companies. They did not, she replied. Burton handed the floor to anti-aging physician Steven Hotze and holistic medicine practitioner David Brownstein. Hotze's patient, Vicki Reynolds, described how 40 years of hormone-induced hell had ended when she took bio-identical hormones. "My family can tolerate me. I don't feel the need to strangle people at any moment," she said. "And I hope that this option is never taken away from me." Burton listened to them all without interrupting.

The hearing drew to a close with a discussion among the panelists, and Burton asked Fugh-Berman again to disclose her funding sources—seemingly convinced she was a spokeswoman for big pharma. "I am really flattered," the professor replied sarcastically. "I do a lot of work against pharmaceutical companies. . . . I'm normally seen as this sort of nuts and granola, herbs and dietary supplement person, so this is a very interesting position for me to be in." Hotze, a former internist who ran an anti-aging clinic in Texas, suggested Fugh-Berman might feel better if she tried anti-aging hormones. "I invite you to come to our office in Houston, be worked up, be evaluated, do a two-month trial and see how you feel." Quipped Fugh-Berman in response, "Thank you. It's going to save me $3,000." She didn't take Hotze up on his offer.

Undaunted by her congressional dressing-down, Fugh-Berman began writing a paper that refuted the marketing claims made for bio-identicals. It was, at times, a solitary mission, which she pursued from a ramshackle Dupont Circle office with caved-in ceilings and no hot water. She surrounded herself with books written by anti-aging doctors, including

Hotze's own *Hormones, Health, and Happiness.* She marked in-
accuracies with Post-it notes, occasionally throwing the books
across the room in frustration. In 2007, she scored a small
coup, getting the paper published in the *Journal of General Internal Medicine.* At the end, she implored the FDA to require
that compounding pharmacists give patients the same warnings about hormones that accompany commercial drugs. "To
do otherwise risks the health of consumers," she wrote in the
article, titled "Bio-identical Hormones for Menopausal Hormone Therapy: Variation on a Theme."

Any suspicions that Fugh-Berman might be shilling for
Wyeth were put to rest by her disclosure at the end of the
paper. In it she revealed that she had served as an expert witness against the company in lawsuits brought by patients who
believed Prempro had given them breast cancer.

The wave of opposition to Premarin and Prempro couldn't have
hit Wyeth at a worse time. When the Women's Health Initiative released its first set of shocking data, the Madison, New
Jersey–based drug giant was still climbing out of a legal quagmire created by fen-phen, the weight-loss drug that it had
pulled from the market in 1997 after some patients developed
heart-valve defects and pulmonary hypertension. The company
would ultimately pay out $19 billion in settlements, making
fen-phen one of the most costly disasters the drug industry had
ever seen. In the wake of the WHI, personal-injury lawyers
pounced again, bringing more than 10,000 cases against Wyeth
that alleged Premarin and Prempro harmed patients.

While Wyeth's lawyers geared up to defend the company's
prized hormone franchise, its scientists took on an entirely

different battle, challenging the anti-aging industry's claims about alternative hormones. It started when Wyeth's vice president for women's health, Ginger Constantine, walked into her local pharmacy to fill a prescription and stumbled on some pamphlets advertising bio-identical hormones. "I was astounded," recalled Constantine, who worked in the company's Collegeville, Pennsylvania, branch office. "They said the products were safer." When she brought the materials in to show her colleagues, they weren't surprised. They, too, had found ads for bio-identicals at their local pharmacies.

Constantine didn't consider herself much of a warrior. A rheumatologist by training, the slight, bespectacled physician was most comfortable talking science with her team or decoding the intricacies of experimental drugs before large audiences of Wall Street analysts. But by 2005, the anti-horse-estrogen propaganda had become too much for her to handle. Constantine's husband was an endocrinologist, and he started to receive promotional newsletters from compounding pharmacists at their home. "There was an onslaught of this following the WHI," Constantine said. "I think the market became really ripe for this to happen."

So Wyeth decided to fight back through the most public forum the drug industry has—the FDA. On October 6, 2005, the company filed a "citizen petition" asking the FDA to take action against compounding pharmacists making homegrown hormones, in order to better protect public health. The 36-page petition alleged that some pharmacies were violating federal laws by mass-marketing their bio-identical hormones and that they were dispensing the drugs with misleading or inadequate safety information. "These pharmacies' failure to provide this legally required information demonstrates forcefully that they are simply trying to dupe an unsuspecting patient population," the petition read. Wyeth was particularly critical of compounded estriol products. The company requested that the FDA confiscate unapproved hormones, or at least issue warning letters to the pharmacies making them.

But Wyeth made a mistake that the anti-aging industry would capitalize on for years to come. The company did not admit in its FDA petition that it was selling its own estriol-based menopause remedy, called Cyclo-Menorette, in four countries: Estonia, Germany, Latvia, and Poland. By failing to disclose its own history with estriol, Wyeth created a perceived conflict of interest. It gave anti-aging doctors and pharmacists a powerful argument: This profit-hungry company, they told patients, wasn't trying to protect public health so much as it was trying to keep a monopoly on the market for all menopause remedies, including estriol.

Wyeth's petition, which the FDA posted on its Web site, unleashed a torrent of responses unlike anything the agency had seen before. Pharmacists, doctors, medical societies, and patients all weighed in, flooding the agency with 70,000 letters. Most blasted Wyeth for trying to beat down their bio-identicals. "Please do not let 'big pharma' take this away," begged Sandra Swert, who informed the agency that after taking bio-identical hormones for eight months, her cholesterol dropped from 225 to 186, her bone density improved, and she no longer needed to take pills for her insomnia and anxiety. Wrote patient Vicki Hedtke, "I have been using bio-identical hormones from a compounding pharmacy to counter menopause issues with no problem. Why is it presumed that if it's made by a multi-national corporation, it's like a commandment from God?"

The responsibility for handling Wyeth's petition was handed to the FDA's office of compliance and its young assistant director, Steven Silverman. He knew he had a sensitive and complex task ahead of him. The chronically understaffed agency only had about a dozen people available to monitor the nation's 3,500 compounding pharmacies. "There are too many pharmacies engaged in too many activities for us to have an absolutely transparent picture of what it is they're producing, and what they're saying about what they're producing at any given time," Silverman conceded.

Silverman's tiny team embarked on a deliberately painstaking research mission. They combed the Internet for misleading claims about compounded hormone products, scrutinized studies of hormone therapies, and sent field agents out to inspect compounding pharmacies throughout the country. They focused much of their attention on estriol, the estrogen subtype that wasn't an ingredient of any FDA-approved drug. What they found concerned Silverman. A scan of the medical literature uncovered 47 estriol studies involving 2,200 patients. "A total of almost 200 adverse events were reported," Silverman said. "Of those, 13 were serious, and one death was reported." In 2006, the FDA collected and tested nearly 200 samples from compounding pharmacies, most of which were finished hormones or chemicals used to make them. Only 33 estrogen and progesterone drugs were hardy enough to withstand the testing process. Nine of those hormones were either too potent, not potent enough, or inconsistent from dose to dose.

More than three years after Wyeth filed its petition, in January 2008, the FDA finally responded. The agency posted an educational brochure on its Web site, *Bio-Identicals: Sorting*

Myths from Facts. The agency listed a number of untruths, dismissing the claims that hormone therapies can be tailored based on saliva samples, that estriol is safer than the other estrogens, and that bio-identical hormones can cure heart disease, Alzheimer's disease, or breast cancer. It recommended that all women take the lowest effective dose of any hormone—compounded or not—for the shortest period of time possible.

The FDA also sent warning letters to seven pharmacies, scolding them for making claims about bio-identical hormones that weren't supported by medical evidence. The pharmacists were warned to stop making products containing estriol and were told if they didn't shape up, they would risk further enforcement, including seizures of the offending drugs. "Each of these pharmacies in our view was engaged in serious misconduct," said Silverman, a lawyer who began his career at the FDA in 2003, in the office of the chief counsel. "They were making uniformly serious misrepresentations about the capacity of their compounded hormone drugs to prevent or treat a variety of diseases, including cancer, Alzheimer's, and stroke."

At Wyeth's women's-health outpost in rural Pennsylvania, Constantine reacted to the FDA's long-awaited response with a tinge of resignation. "I think they probably did the best they could do," she said, noting that the agency's reach was somewhat limited by its scant resources and lack of power over individual pharmacies. Pausing to search for a bright spot in the three-year ordeal, she pointed out that several medical organizations, including the Endocrine Society and the American College of Obstetricians and Gynecologists, followed the FDA's lead and issued public statements discouraging the use of bio-identical hormones.

The pioneer of bio-identicals wasn't about to let the drug industry have the final word, however. After the FDA responded to Wyeth's petition, Jonathan Wright partnered with several alternative-medicine nonprofits to form a group they dubbed the Hands Off My Estrogens! (HOME) Coalition. They scraped together enough money to place a one-page ad in the *New York Times* and three other major publications on February 4, 2008. "FDA Bans Hormone Produced by Human Body as 'Unapproved' Drug," blared the ad's headline. "Act now to defend your right to bio-identical hormones!" In two full columns of small type, Wright spelled out all the claims about estriol that he had spent the last two decades preaching so effectively: It's safe because pregnant women make lots of it; drug companies don't offer it because they can't patent it; there have been no adverse events linked to it. He accused the FDA of pandering to "its clients," the drug industry. "Fees from the big drug companies pay for a sizeable share of the FDA's budget and staff," he wrote.

Anti-aging proponents claimed Wyeth sold estriol all over Europe and that it was a major supplier of raw estriol to other companies. At anti-aging conferences and training sessions, they sniped about Wyeth's monopolistic and underhanded attempts to protect its own products. In June 2008, an advocacy group calling itself the American Association for Health Freedom joined the effort, shelling out more than $20,000 to place two full-page color ads in *Roll Call*, a newspaper for Capitol Hill insiders. The ads urged readers to support House Resolution 342 and Senate Resolution 88, both of which sought to reverse the FDA's estriol restrictions. "Shame on you, Wyeth," the ads said, admonishing the drug giant for supposedly promoting its estriol product in Europe as "an ideal therapy" for menopause.

"Why is bio-identical estriol ideal for European women but un-safe for American women?" They reveled in news that Wyeth had reimbursed *Feminine Forever* author Robert Wilson for ex-penses he had incurred while writing his book on Premarin. Two decades after Wilson's death, his son told the *New York Times* that the drug company had also donated money to the Wilson Research Foundation and paid him to lecture to women's groups around the country about the wonders of hor-mone replacement.

A4M's Pamela Smith cheerily chimed in on the Wyeth bash-ing. She heard that estriol was being tested to treat multiple sclerosis (MS) and latched on to the news as the latest proof that estriol was a safe and effective treatment for women. When asked who might be developing that drug, she said, "I would look for Wyeth Corporation being the one doing it, be-cause they're the ones making it in Europe."

Although Wyeth was studying remedies to treat multiple sclerosis, none of its experimental drugs were made of estriol. There was one large trial of estriol in MS patients in the United States, sponsored by the National Multiple Sclerosis Society, which received grants from several drug companies, including Wyeth. But no company provided direct funding for the estriol study, and the research wasn't expected to be completed before 2013. During the two decades that Wyeth sold estriol, it mar-keted the product only to gynecologists—not directly to pa-tients. No one at the company had any recollection of using the terminology "ideal therapy" to describe estriol. And Wyeth didn't sell raw estriol to other companies, a spokesman said.

In the end, Cyclo-Menorette performed so poorly that Wyeth axed the product just a few months after filing its com-plaint on bio-identical hormones to the FDA. Its revenues from all the drugs it sold in Estonia, Germany, Latvia, and Poland were so small the company didn't even bother breaking them out for investors. All told, the anti-aging industry's argument that Wyeth was only trying to protect its own interest in estriol was nonsense. By 2008, Wyeth had written estriol off as useless. "I think it is just so weak," Constantine said. As for congressional resolutions 342 and 88, they stalled on the Hill while legislators grappled with more pressing issues, like the failing economy and the war in Iraq.

The FDA's Silverman said he would welcome any evidence that estriol was safe, regardless of what disease was being studied or who did the studying. "If there were an FDA-approved drug that contained estriol, then the concern that pharmacists were compounding using an active ingredient that wasn't part of an approved drug would disappear," he said. But the agency would still be troubled that the safety and efficacy of estriol as a menopause remedy had not been proven, he added.

In spite of the FDA's warnings—and even as a flood of studies confirmed that hormones could be carcinogenic—patients ran to their corner pharmacies, toting their custom-designed prescriptions for compounded bio-identical estrogen and progesterone. Anti-aging doctors and pharmacists fed into the frenzy by pointing to Wyeth's bad behavior as the prime example of why natural hormones were so much safer than drugs made by big bad pharma. In 2009, lawyers representing patients who believed they had been harmed by Prempro uncovered more than 30 examples of favorable articles about the drug that were produced by Wyeth-paid ghostwriters—further proof, anti-aging proponents said, that the pharmaceutical industry was putting profits before patients' best interests. Wyeth's sales of Premarin and Prempro fell from $2.1 billion in 2001 to under a billion dollars a year.

Meanwhile, in the year following its response to Wyeth's petition, the FDA received 26 reports of adverse events from patients taking compounded estriol, including 10 reports of breast cancer. But it had yet to seize any bio-identical hormones from any compounding pharmacy.

CHAPTER 5

The Hollywood Connection

In 2004, millions of women started taking medical advice from the most unlikely source: Suzanne Somers, the actress who played Chrissy Snow on *Three's Company*. In a book called *The Sexy Years*, Somers wrote about her struggles against "The Seven Dwarfs of Menopause," whom she dubbed "Itchy," "Bitchy," "Sweaty," "Sleepy," "Bloated," "Forgetful," and "All Dried Up." The cure, she declared, was bio-identical hormones, or as she put it, "the elixir—the juice of youth that has sent the Seven Dwarfs of Menopause off to the coal mines never to return!" Her timing couldn't have been better. Millions of women had just abandoned Premarin and Prempro and were looking for alternatives to help them survive menopause. They snapped up Somers's book, toted it to their ob-gyns, and demanded prescriptions for the natural hormones that the actress told them were just like the ones their own bodies used to make. When their doctors refused, they turned to anti-aging clinics instead.

It seems inconceivable that a medical phenomenon could be so influenced by a washed-up TV star. This was, after all, the woman who was best known for snorting when she laughed and for spouting lines like "I love surprises—funny how you never expect them." But this was no fad. Five years after Somers wrote about her bio-identical awakening, Oprah Winfrey invited her to appear on *The Oprah Winfrey Show* as a menopause expert. Winfrey had recently discovered bio-identical hormones, and she was so enamored of them that she decided to open "a national conversation on hormone-replacement therapy," she told viewers, with two shows and a story in her monthly magazine, *O*. In January 2009, Somers sat across from Winfrey on her Chicago soundstage and declared, "I feel better at 62 than I ever have in my whole life." Winfrey cut to a video of Somers demonstrating her daily regimen of bio-identical estradiol, estriol, and progesterone. Somers rubbed the creams into her arms and sat at her kitchen table with a lineup of 60 supplement pills she planned to take that day. "Many people write Suzanne Somers off as a quackadoo," Winfrey joked. "But she just might be a pioneer."

Nine hundred miles away from Winfrey's Chicago soundstage, Nancy Chapman was driving from her home in Westerly, Rhode Island, to Manchester, Connecticut, for a follow-up appointment with anti-aging doctor Alicia Stanton. Chapman went through menopause late, at age 58. After her longtime doctor said her dark moods and sleeplessness were no big deal, she sought out Stanton, who was the chief medical officer of BodyLogicMD, a chain of 25 anti-aging centers. Stanton put Chapman on an extensive hormone-replacement plan that included bio-identical progesterone and estrogen, plus testosterone injections every other week to spice up her sex drive.

"I'm 100 percent better," Chapman told the doctor. "My energy is much better. I have fewer mood swings. I'm thinking about sex for once. It's fantastic." Chapman wasn't even aware of anti-aging medicine until she read *The Sexy Years*. "That got me started on this," said Chapman, a distinguished-looking woman with groomed blond hair and black-rimmed glasses perched on the end of her nose. "Suzanne Somers is a terrific promoter."

While Stanton consulted with Chapman at a small conference table in her office, the phones rang nonstop in the background. "I'm booked until May," said Stanton, breathlessly juggling office visits and phone calls, while she sucked on a Dunkin' Donuts coffee. BodyLogic started the year totally caught up on prospects. "That was before the Oprah factor," Stanton said. "Now we're 2,000 patients behind." In January, BodyLogic fielded calls from 7,115 prospective patients—more than 900 of whom signed on to become customers. "That was a 300 percent increase from December," said Stanton, who herself was fielding more than 40 inquiries a day from patients willing to drive for hours to see her.

With *The Sexy Years*, Somers legitimized anti-aging medicine in a way that Klatz and practitioners like Stanton had been unable to achieve. And the actress did it by perpetuating myths about hormone therapy. She started the book by proudly recounting her 2000 battle against breast cancer, which she said she had won by rejecting chemotherapy and continuing to use her bio-identical hormones, even though her doctors begged her to stop taking them. "Women are deprived of their hormones when they have cancer because it is thought to be safer, legally, to take them off hormones *in case* hormones feed tumors," Somers wrote. "Also, I knew most doctors thought of 'hormones' as the synthetic type, which are not really hormones at all." Only a few pages in, Somers had already declared that there was no link between bio-identicals and cancer. Readers may not have realized that Somers had started taking bio-identical hormones well before she developed breast cancer.

Somers paved a golden path for the anti-aging industry—one that allowed doctors to fabricate a distinction between drug-company hormones and bio-identicals made by compounding pharmacists. "Because we are living longer than ever before, the new thinking is to *replace* the hormones lost in the aging process. This *cannot* be done with the synthetic hormones put out by the drug companies," Somers wrote. "Only natural bio-identical hormones can do that, because they are made from plant extracts and exactly mimic the hormones we make naturally in our bodies." She didn't explain that drug companies made bio-identicals, too, and furthermore that they produced them in federally monitored factories. Nor did she inform patients that they could purchase FDA-approved bio-identicals through their HMOs and at regular pharmacies.

Throughout the book, Somers sprinkled in interviews with physicians such as Diana Schwarzbein, the Santa Barbara, California, endocrinologist who first turned Somers on to bio-identicals. To relieve her menopause symptoms, Somers began taking estrogen and progesterone "cyclically"—estrogen every day, and progesterone the last two weeks of the month. That way, she would menstruate once a month, mimicking the periods she'd had before menopause. She was convinced that that's what nature intended. In *The Sexy Years*, Schwarzbein explained that drugs like Premarin were problems not just because of their "synthetic" origins but also because of how they were prescribed. "Unfortunately, by messing with Mother Nature and giving drug hormones without restoring menstrual bleeding, we have done more harm than good," Schwarzbein said. "You have to have a period, because this mimics normal!" She said that it was safe for women to take bio-identicals their whole lives, as long as "we keep adjusting the amount to match your ever-changing lifestyle." Neither she nor Somers provided references to any scientific studies showing that hormones can be taken safely, either cyclically or not, for decades on end.

Some of Somers's interviews in *The Sexy Years* were so nutty they might as well have been pulled verbatim from *Three's Company*. "Why are there no sexual medications for women?" Somers asked Laura Berman, a sex therapist and frequent TV personality. "Until several years ago, women were not allowed to be included in any clinical trials," Berman replied erroneously. Somers bought it, however, and replied, "Why—are our genitals not as important?"

Early in the book, ob-gyn Uzzi Reiss propagated the anti–big pharma sentiment that would prove so essential to furthering the anti-aging mythology. Somers asked Reiss, "Why are we not giving women hormones that are an exact replica?" Reiss answered, "Because natural bio-identical hormones cannot be patented." But even Reiss tripped over the distinction between synthetic and natural. "Only bio-identical HRT [hormone-replacement therapy]," he told Somers, "synthesized in a lab, made from plant extracts, exactly replicates what our bodies make." How can something that's synthesized in a lab be less synthetic than a drug made in a factory? Somers was obviously unaware of the non sequitur.

Despite Somers's unabashed disgust for drug-company commercialism, she set up her entire book as a promotional vehicle for anti-aging products—some of which, oddly enough, were made by pharmaceutical companies. Pfizer's Viagra got a plug as an effective sexual aid for women, as did AndroGel, a testosterone product made by Solvay Pharmaceuticals. Interviewee Berman directed women to her Web site, which sold a colorful collection of sex toys such as "The Adonis," an appropriately named vibrator. *The Sexy Years* ended with a six-page list of anti-aging doctors and pharmacies, complete with phone numbers and Web addresses.

The Sexy Years spent 25 weeks on the *New York Times* list of best-selling advice books.

The story of how Somers chose to use her celebrity firepower to combat hot flashes and dull sex drives is one she related without a hint of compunction. It started at her 50th birthday party in 1996, she said, when her son, Bruce, got up to deliver a toast. "He started to say things like, 'You are my life, Ma,' and I couldn't hear what he was saying because I was so hot. I kept on saying to everybody, 'Are you hot? Oh my God, I'm so hot,'" Somers recalled in a phone interview. "And that was the beginning of my menopausal symptoms." Somers spent the next three years shuttling from doctor to doctor. She was offered everything from Prozac, to control her moods, to painkillers, to relieve her joint pain. "I asked the last traditional doctor I saw, 'Is this the best you have to offer women?' He patted me on the back and said, 'The drug companies know best, dear.' So that's when I realized was on my own."

The sitcom star's homage to hormones was so successful she wrote two follow-up books, *Ageless* and *Breakthrough*. Anti-aging doctors and pharmacists devoured the collection, turning the books into their own personal marketing tools. After New York doctor Rashmi Gulati scored a brief mention in *Age-*

less, she tacked a photo of herself with the actress on her Web site. Then Gulati bought a sponsored link on Google so that when patients searched for "bio-identical hormones," her home page popped up at the top of the search results, with the headline "Suzanne Somers Recommends."

West Hollywood anti-aging physician Gary London got such a huge boost in business that in 2006 he felt compelled to express his appreciation by writing his own book and titling it *Thank You Suzanne Somers*. London started the book with a letter he wrote to Somers applauding her for *The Sexy Years*. "It was so honest and clear and compelling that it introduced a huge audience to an exciting new world where vitality can outlast youth," London wrote. London, an ob-gyn who started practicing anti-aging medicine full-time in 2005, explained that as soon as his book came out, he started getting calls from actors and studio executives, some as young as 35. "They felt they were not at their peak, and they wanted to get back to where they were," London said. "Suddenly everybody was talking about hormones. Somers was the salesman."

After Oprah Winfrey promoted Somers from quackadoo to anti-aging prophet, BodyLogicMD made the most of the free PR. Its Web site boasted that BodyLogic had been listed as a resource in Somers's books and on Oprah Winfrey's Web site (www.Oprah.com). Stanton posted a glowing press release on BodyLogic's Web site, declaring, "I applaud Oprah on her willingness to initiate this conversation with America. There is so much more to discuss!" Two months later, BodyLogic physician Stephen Center held a seminar on hormone replacement in his San Diego office. Nearly 20 people, most of them women, showed up, filing into Center's small waiting room, which he packed with folding chairs and a projector that shined PowerPoint slides on the wall. He put three handouts on each chair, including an offer for free blood and saliva tests (a $500 value!) for anyone who referred three patients to his office.

The doctor, who spoke at rapid-fire speed, asked for a show of hands. How many had seen Suzanne Somers on *Oprah*? Five hands shot up. One woman hadn't seen the show but had heard about it from her friends, so she went to Winfrey's Web site. She clicked over to BodyLogic's site from there and decided to attend Center's seminar so she could find out more. "Well I'm at, you know, *that age*," said the 40-something woman, eliciting a quiet chorus of "uh-huhs" and chuckles from people in neighboring seats. Each attendee got a follow-up phone call and e-mail, offering answers to any questions and help scheduling a BodyLogic appointment. Center said Winfrey's shows immediately drove up traffic to his office. "Oprah's been very good to us. I praise her every day."

But while BodyLogic was publicly celebrating the newfound exposure for anti-aging medicine, privately Alicia Stanton was dealing with the confusion it wrought in some patients. One of her patients called her and asked if it was really safe to stay on bio-identical hormones indefinitely. "My opinion is, if they continue to be balanced, you should be on them indefinitely," Stanton responded. A moment later, the patient asked the question again. "I just want to do the right thing," she said. "I'm concerned about whether it's safe." Said Stanton, "It's up to you. If you want to wind down, you can. A lot of people are on them indefinitely."

A woman attending Center's seminar e-mailed him afterward to ask why he didn't prescribe the FDA-approved bio-identical hormones Vivelle and Climara, which were likely to be covered by most patients' insurance plans. "Vivelle and Climara are not bio-identical," he e-mailed back. She replied, "Climara is derived from soy; Vivelle is derived from yams. Why are they not considered bio-identical?" Center explained that those products only contained estradiol, and that BodyLogic's standard policy was to prescribe compounded combinations of hormones containing 80 percent estriol and 20 percent estradiol, "roughly mimicking the same ratio as in nature."

What that could mean was that BodyLogic's doctors were urging women to get blood and saliva tests to measure their hormone levels but were not necessarily tailoring the prescriptions to match the results of those tests. Instead, it appeared that for many patients they were recommending an 80/20 estrogen mix that was heavily weighted toward the most tepid form of the hormone—estriol. When queried about this, BodyLogic's chief medical officer, Stanton, claimed that doctors might use different percentages as patients' needs dictated. Contradicting Center's statement, Stanton said, "We also use commercially available bio-identical estradiol patches."

But patients couldn't even meet a BodyLogic doctor without first getting their blood and saliva tested by the company's laboratory-testing partner. And rather than encouraging patients to save money by buying FDA-approved estradiol through their health plans, BodyLogic doctors often suggested patients buy compounded hormones through the company's pharmacy partners.

That might have had something to do with BodyLogic's business model. When asked how the company made most of its money, said CEO Patrick Savage, "I make it off the labs that are ordered and the vitamins, supplements and products." BodyLogic had "business agreements" with outside companies

that provided those products and services. That set up a potential conflict of interest—and one patients might not have
known about.

The stronger the Hollywood endorsement of hormones grew,
the more acceptable it became for anti-aging doctors to prescribe them in particularly high doses. BodyLogic's Stanton was
among hundreds of physicians in the United States who sometimes prescribed estrogen and progesterone according to regimens designed by T. S. Wiley, a California woman whom
Somers featured as an expert hormone clinician in *Ageless*.
Wiley believed that every woman could achieve eternal youth
by ratcheting her hormone levels back up to those of a 20-year-
old and cycling them in tandem with the lunar calendar, taking
the highest doses of estrogen when the moon was at its fullest
and adding progesterone in the final two weeks of the month.

Wiley introduced her unconventional protocol to the world
in 2003 in a book she called *Sex, Lies, and Menopause: The Shocking Truth About Synthetic Hormones and the Benefits of Natural Alternatives*. She recommended women take between 8 and 16
milligrams a day of estradiol, and between 200 and 700 milligrams a day of progesterone. To understand how big a hormone overdose that is, consider that Climara delivered just 0.1
milligram a day of estradiol at its highest dose. And the FDA-
approved progesterone Prometrium was rarely prescribed at
more than 400 milligrams a day. Yet Wiley downplayed the
discrepancy in her book, stressing that bio-identicals were
natural and coaching readers on how to appease any doctor
who was reluctant to prescribe such high doses. "Remind him

of 'all young women'—that is, if high episodic doses of estrogen caused cancer, all young women would be dead," Wiley wrote.

Wiley's doses were even more aggressive than those common in the days of *Feminine Forever*, when doctors prescribed Premarin at doses of 1.25–2.5 milligrams per day. (Today's recommended dose is no more than 1.25 milligrams.) But Wiley, a gruff woman who often mocked her critics, scoffed at concerns that her protocol was too aggressive. "When a woman wants to take hormones, the 800-pound gorilla in the room is cancer. I came to believe none of that," Wiley said. "My conclusion was that they control cancer, not cause it."

Few paid attention to Wiley until *Ageless* was published in 2006. Somers introduced Wiley as "an anthropologist focusing on evolutionary biology and environmental endocrinology in molecular medicine and genetics" and as "a member of the New York Academy of Sciences." In the printed interview with Wiley, Somers revealed that a few years after her bout with cancer, she had developed endometrial hyperplasia, a precancerous condition marked by excessive growth of the uterine wall and bleeding. Somers's doctors persuaded her to have a hysterectomy to prevent uterine cancer. That was the standard of care for hyperplasia, but Wiley wasn't buying it. Instead, she blamed Somers's illness on stem cells—the body's "master cells," which possess the ability to change into any tissue or organ in the body but have never been universally implicated in cancer. "The stem cells in your breast made some wonky cells, and we'll call them cancer," Wiley said. "But the stem cell in your leg can make breast cancer because a stem cell anywhere can make anything. That's how *I* believe metastasis occurs." She went on to declare, "If women were given hormones rhythmically, I believe very few would need to have their uteruses removed." When Somers told Wiley that doctors blame excessive bleeding on too much estrogen, Wiley replied, "Sorry, they're wrong."

Little did readers know that Wiley didn't have a degree in any science, not even anthropology. After press reports questioned her claim that she had earned a bachelor's from Webster University in 1975, critics noted, she changed the biography on her Web site to read "Pending B.A. in Anthropology." She later removed any reference to her education. She had never earned the degree. As for her membership in the New York Academy of Sciences, anyone can get one of those—for $108 a year.

Wiley's recommendations were so high that even the staunchest supporters of bio-identical hormones scrambled to distance themselves from her. A4M's Pamela Smith refused to teach the Wiley Protocol to anti-aging doctors. The whole idea flew in the face of what anti-aging medicine was about, she said, and "the dosages were dramatically high." Jonathan Wright, the pioneer of bio-identical estrogen, put it more bluntly: "This woman is out there advocating enormous doses of estradiol. Well that is DUMBDY-DUMB-DUMB."

Some of the doctors who appeared in *Ageless* were mortified to learn that Wiley would be in the book, too. Erika Schwartz, a Manhattan-based anti-aging doctor and TV personality, had come across the Wiley Protocol several years earlier when her agent had begged her to prescribe the high hormone doses. Schwartz, who goes by the nickname "Dr. Erika," was quoted only briefly in *Ageless*, but she wanted out of it altogether. So she called Somers's agent on the eve of the book's October 2006 release. "I said, 'Listen, I would like to go on record that if Wiley's in the book, I would like my name removed from the book.' I'm not gonna give credibility to somebody who I think is out of her mind, basically," said Schwartz, a native Romanian whose news-anchor looks and enthusiasm for youth extension scored her a gig on the entertainment news show *Extra*.

When *Ageless* was released as planned, Schwartz and six other doctors dashed off a scathing letter to Somers's editor at Crown Publishing, a unit of Random House. "Wiley has no medical or clinical qualifications," they wrote. "To our dismay, Wiley dispenses gratuitous advice on significant medical issues including the use of bio-identical hormone therapies, areas that are legally and ethically the domain of licensed medical practitioners." Among the cosigners was Diana Schwarzbein, the doctor who first introduced Somers to anti-aging medicine.

The letter caught the attention of CNN's Larry King, who invited Somers, Schwarzbein, Schwartz, and Wiley to appear on his show *Larry King Live* on November 15. An all-out catfight ensued. Somers said Schwarzbein and Schwartz hadn't even read *Ageless* before they wrote their protest letter. "I read every word of the book," Schwartz said. "No you didn't. No you didn't," Somers insisted. Schwartz shot back, "And you know what? This should not be an argument about Suzanne Somers or Wiley. It's about women." King tried to break it up. "Erika, hold on a second," he said. "It's about women's safety," Schwartz cried. King tried again to interject. "Erika, hold it a second." Then Schwarzbein jumped in, reporting that she had received complaints from patients who had been harmed by the Wiley Protocol. Wiley snapped, "And we hold meetings in Santa Barbara once a month for 50 to 80 people on the Wiley Protocol, and it is remarkable how many of them are your ex-patients, Diana."

Wulf Utian of the North American Menopause Society also appeared on the show, but he had barely begun to speak when he was once again blasted for being the mouthpiece of big pharma. "Larry, I think the whole group, as I heard it, are all off base," Utian said. "The physicians, if you go to their Web sites, are selling promises, silver bullets against aging with barely a nanoshred of evidence for proving what they're claiming." Somers couldn't contain herself. "Dr. Utian is funded by Wyeth Pharmaceuticals," she said. "I am not funded by Wyeth Pharmaceuticals. I'm not," Utian shouted back. "I have it in my purse here if you'd like me to bring out more pages," Somers offered. "I Googled you today. Your information is all out there. You're funded by Pfizer and SmithKline." Said King in a desperate attempt to be the voice of reason, "That doesn't make him wrong."

King was smart to deflect the conversation away from the drug industry, but he was too late. Wiley's ascent—along with so many other puzzling anti-aging phenomena—had already been secured. The anti-aging community's maniacal dismissal of anyone with a hint of pharmaceutical funding only helped its cause. Anti-aging fanatics had little trouble convincing patients that drug companies were evil. Some doctors suggested that big pharma paid people to say that compounded hormones were dangerous so they could preserve the market for their own "synthetic" versions. Patients never suspected that synthetic and natural were one and the same and that both could be deadly at high doses. That's why so many women marched willingly into the Wiley Protocol, exposing themselves to doses of hormones that mainstream doctors would immediately recognize were precarious.

To many scientists, the Wiley Protocol was little more than out-and-out abuse disguised as medical research. University of

Kentucky bioethicist M. Sara Rosenthal exposed the protocol as unethical in the November 2008 issue of the *Journal of the North American Menopause Society*. Rosenthal explained that the protocol was described as a clinical trial, even though there was no standardized way to collect data on the women who adhered to it. Therefore, doctors administering the protocol were not obligated to check up on their patients. Furthermore, Rosenthal detailed in her article, the protocol was based on financial relationships among Wiley, her corporation, "Wiley Protocol-registered" compounding pharmacists, and prescribing doctors, in which they stood to gain from attracting new patients—in contravention of conventional clinical trial practices. Wiley allowed pharmacists to "register" as official Wiley Protocol prescribers, but only if they also stocked her book, which guaranteed that she would receive royalty income. "I'm appalled," Rosenthal said. "This is a business purporting to do research. She's taking advantage of vulnerable women who are already uncomfortable with what's happening to their bodies."

Some former Wiley patients tried to warn women away from the program by publicizing their own horror stories about it. Laurel McCubbin started the Wiley Protocol in 2004 and felt great for about two months. But then a cascade of scary symptoms started. "I was bleeding at the wrong times, really extreme bleeding," McCubbin said. "My hair was falling out." During the "luteal" phase, which called for high doses of progesterone, she lost the ability to sleep. "It was progesterone poisoning," McCubbin said. When she called Wiley to ask about the side effects, she was brushed off. "I pressed her for the documentation that we should use this much progesterone," McCubbin said. "She told me I was being ungrateful. When I told her my hair was falling out, she said, 'You need to get your thyroid checked.'"

McCubbin quit the protocol and started a support group for Wiley refugees. They flocked to her Web site, Rhythmic Living (www.rhythmicliving.org), eager to describe their hormone nightmares. One woman ended up in the emergency room with kidney stones. Another gained 25 pounds and developed mysterious dark lines down her belly and above her lip. Yet another got so depressed she couldn't get out of bed for two months. Then she had to have her gall bladder removed. Her surgeon surmised too much estrogen had done it in.

Neither Wiley nor Somers was fazed by the attacks. "It seems like professional envy," Wiley said. "I'm precise. I'm scrupulous. I research something for years. People can see I produce quality research and I only work with scientists and doctors." Somers refused to consider that Wiley's recommendations might be dangerous, and she credited Wiley with turning her on to rhythmic cycling.

Stanton patient Holly Dreher, 61, was following the Wiley Protocol and taking an even bigger dose of estrogen than the program recommended. But when she arrived at Stanton's Manchester office in January 2009, she told the doctor that she'd been suffering from cramps and that her period had come a day early the last time. "Increase the progesterone," Stanton advised her. "I don't like progesterone," replied Dreher, explaining that the hormone made her feel bloated. "So decrease the estrogen," said Stanton. "I can't do that," said Dreher. "I can tell by my symptoms I need a lot of estrogen." She chose to tolerate the side effects instead.

Dreher didn't pay much attention to the experts who said that too much estrogen can cause breast cancer and that not balancing the estrogen with progesterone can endanger the uterus. "When people say you'll get cancer if you take hormones your whole life I don't believe it," said Dreher, a vivacious blond who sought out Stanton after her internist questioned her hormone routine. "I showed him my schedule," she said, pointing to a green calendar, provided by Wiley, detailing the dosages for each day. "His eyes bugged out. He said, 'This is a lot of hormones.' But it's what I need. I have four granddaughters. I can still run around with them. If I stop, I'll be worse, because I'll be older. I read in Suzanne Somers's book that she needs a lot of estrogen." Dreher seemed to understand that she could maintain her youthful energy by exercising and watching her diet, but she preferred the hormone route to youth. "I know it's not natural to be getting a period at my age, but I wanted it. I could give up my wine. I could give up my cookies in the afternoon." She paused, turning to her husband, Mark, who had joined her for the consultation with Stanton. "But you have to enjoy yourself," Mark said. "I don't want to drink alone."

Despite her support for Holly Dreher's massive hormone doses, Stanton seemed to have a gut feeling that Wiley's methodology was flawed. The protocol demanded that women get regular blood tests to measure their hormones, even though hormones given in cream form don't show up in the blood. "I don't completely follow how she gets her numbers," Stanton said. "If you test anyone on a Wiley Protocol by any other method—if you use saliva or urine—their hormone levels are very, very high. But in blood they stay low. I just don't understand." She didn't encourage new patients to try Wiley, but she didn't try to talk women out of the program, either.

Mark Dreher was so impressed with his wife's anti-aging routine that he shelled out $495 for a battery of BodyLogic blood and saliva tests for himself. Stanton told him that the saliva tests revealed abnormally high levels of estrogen; it had clearly rubbed off on him while he was sleeping next to his wife. High estrogen can cause heart trouble in men. Yet Stanton joked, asking Mark if he cried during Hallmark commercials because he had so much more of the "female" hormone than most men did. She told Holly to rinse the cream off her arms before going to bed. "My guess is, it's in the sheets," Stanton said.

Mark Dreher didn't seem like an obvious candidate for anti-aging medicine. At 63, he was trim and active, with blue eyes and a full head of brown hair. He took vitamins and fish oil, never smoked, ate sensibly, and listed his only vices as five cups of coffee and two glasses of wine per day. "I feel sorry for people who don't feel good," he told Stanton, adding that he might hit the snooze button in the morning but usually bounded out of bed by 7 a.m. He shyly hinted to Stanton that he would like to improve his and Holly's sex life. "Pump it up," he joked. "I just want it to be better." Stanton told him his testosterone level was that of an 80-year-old man, and she immediately prescribed a regimen of testosterone gel and DHEA capsules. (Dehydroepiandrosterone, or DHEA, is a "precursor hormone"; it is made by the adrenal glands and then converts to sex hormones such as testosterone.)

The story of how Stanton got to this place—a once-sought-after ob-gyn, now endorsing extensive hormone regimens—is a study in how the anti-aging industry was built. Growing up in Elmira, New York, Stanton was the brainy kid who performed surgery on her Barbie Dolls rather than dressing them in frilly outfits. After graduating with honors from the State University of New York at Buffalo in 1990, she built a leading ob-gyn practice in Hartford, Connecticut, with 8,000 patients and 16 employees. Then, in October 1997, at the age of 34, she was diagnosed with a spinal cord tumor. "I was told I'd be dead by Christmas," the doctor recalled. Surgeons removed the tumor successfully and declared her cancer-free. But she lost most of the feeling in her right leg, making it impossible to deliver babies or perform surgery. So she decided to specialize in hormone therapy and alternative medicine.

Then patients started bringing Stanton copies of *The Sexy Years*. She was fascinated. She attended some A4M conferences and signed up for the seminars on bio-identical hormone replacement. "I looked at the biochemistry and the way physiology works, and I was like, ahhh," she said with a gasp. "It's so cool. How can people not get this?" Stanton began trying bio-identical hormones on patients who didn't respond to traditional therapies. She was so amazed by the results that she closed her practice and went into anti-aging medicine full-time in 2005.

Knowing her patients would be paying out of pocket for her hormone recipes, Stanton considered setting up shop in upscale Glastonbury, Connecticut. Then she met Deborah Ravenwood, a part-time pet therapist who was looking for a business partner to bring more traffic to her holistic medicine center in middle-class Manchester. Stanton set up her practice in a small, homey cabin just across the walk from Paws and Listen, where Ravenwood counseled pet owners with psychotic cats and destructive dogs. The decidedly unmedical look of the place didn't dissuade patients from driving vast distances, sometimes more than two hours from Boston or New York, to see Stanton.

For the young physician, anti-aging medicine proved a remarkably easy way to earn more money than doctors of her generation had come to expect. As an ob-gyn, she billed $1.3 million a year but cleared only $150,000. The HMOs undercut her on every procedure she billed, and her malpractice insurance cost $65,000 a year. After she joined BodyLogic in 2005, she started pulling in up to 15 new patients a week, each of whom paid $395 cash for an initial one-hour appointment. Stanton collected $275 for follow-up appointments and $150 for phone consultations. She said goodbye to the hassles of HMOs and was able to buy a basic liability policy for a mere $10,000 a year.

After Suzanne Somers's *Ageless* was published in 2006, Stanton was invited to have dinner at the actress's Palm Springs, California, home, along with 50 or so other anti-aging luminaries. Built on the side of a hill, the house had a trolley that shuttled guests to the front door. Thousands of candles illuminated the back patio, where Stanton sat at a table with T. S. Wiley. The flap over *Ageless* dampened neither the festive mood nor the welcoming of Wiley into the anti-aging club. "I have a lot of respect for what [Wiley] has to say," Stanton said. "She's a brilliant woman."

Somers may have introduced anti-aging hormones to droves of dried-up women, but it was Oprah Winfrey who escorted the creams into the realm of mainstream medicine. During the first of her two shows on the topic, Winfrey told her audience that she had terrible insomnia during menopause, but her doctor said that her hormone levels were in the normal range. "But normal for whom?" Winfrey asked. "There are legions of women . . . walking around feeling like crap." She featured Robin McGraw, wife of TV's Dr. Phil, the psychologist Winfrey had turned into a star a decade earlier. Robin McGraw described her experience with bio-identicals, which she had written about in a new book, *What's Age Got to Do with It?* McGraw introduced her doctor, Los Angeles–based Prudence Hall, whose practice revolved around prescribing bio-identical estrogen, progesterone, and testosterone at levels she believed would bring patients back to age 35.

Winfrey's producers had also talked to Utian, but they ran less than two minutes of the taped interview during the show. "There's no such thing as a natural hormone," Utian said, repeating warnings about compounded hormones that he had tried to get across so many times before. If you believe they're safer, he said, "you believe in the tooth fairy."

Throughout the show, Winfrey chatted via the Internet videophone Skype with a patient she called Michelle, broadcasting their conversation on a huge video screen behind the stage. Michelle, a dowdy 45-year-old Canadian with a strained voice, was miserable with hot flashes and insomnia. "It is hell. Literally burning hell," she said. So Winfrey gave her a parting gift: a visit to Dr. Hall, with Robin McGraw as her escort.

Was this about helping women, or was it about selling books and encouraging viewers to pay exorbitant fees to anti-aging doctors and pharmacists? To many mainstream doctors watching the show, it looked like the latter. Winfrey vowed to take a balanced approach to hormone replacement, and her history of dealing with controversial topics suggested she would be fair. But during the second show, Somers sat on the stage across from Winfrey, while two ob-gyns were relegated to seats in the audience, where they were expected to sit quietly until called upon to speak. They were Christiane Northrup, author of *The Wisdom of Menopause*, and Lauren Streicher, assistant professor of Obstetrics and Gynecology at Northwestern University. Winfrey exclaimed, "We have the right to demand a better quality of life for ourselves!" As the audience applauded, Somers celebrated her triumph over the Seven Dwarfs of Menopause, telling the mostly female crowd, "The more of us who are hormonally balanced, the better the planet will be."

The camera panned often to Somers's 71-year-old husband, Alan Hamel. "He looks good," Winfrey said. "He's on testosterone," Somers replied.

Northwestern physician Streicher wasn't opposed to prescribing bio-identicals, provided they were FDA approved. But she felt strongly that women had been misled into believing that they were safer than other hormones. Streicher had been a vocal opponent of Somers ever since the publication of *The Sexy Years*, criticizing the actress in a column in the *Chicago Sun Times* and appearing on TV news shows to debate her. A few of Winfrey's producers were Streicher's patients, and they invited her to appear on the show with Somers. Streicher asked whether she would be able to sit on the stage with Winfrey and was reassured that she would. So she ordered up a copy of Somers's third book, *Breakthrough,* on her Kindle electronic reader and made notes on the screen every time she found an inaccuracy. "The notes got to be longer than the book. It was ridiculous," Streicher recalled.

Somers wasn't thrilled to hear that her nemesis would be on the show. And a few weeks before the taping, Winfrey's producers told Streicher she'd have to sit in the audience. "It was not acceptable to sit there and have to respond to Dr. Somers," Streicher said. "It made her the expert and put me in the defensive spot. Suddenly I was the witch who didn't want women to feel good."

But Streicher went anyway, sitting on the edge of her chair and talking rapidly so she could have all her major points heard. "Whether you go to your corner drugstore or your compounding pharmacy, you're most likely to get an estrogen that was synthesized," Streicher said. "'Bio-identical' is a made-up term. Marketers made it up. It sounds really catchy." Winfrey jumped in: "We might as well use the word now because it's out there, OK?" Said Streicher, "It's out there but it's a problem, because the implication is that it's something safer, it's something better, it's something different. Chemically the structure is exactly the same." The patient Michelle, who appeared on Skype again—this time with a new haircut and blond highlights—soon upstaged Streicher. She had only been on bio-identicals for nine days, but she said she felt better than she had ever remembered feeling before. "The side effect from the bio-identicals is a big dose of joy," she gushed.

After Streicher reluctantly played Wicked Witch to Somers's Snow White, she returned to her office and was stunned to find that 300 patients had called during the show to request appointments. Many of them believed they had been harmed by bio-identicals. One woman was diagnosed with breast cancer, underwent a bilateral mastectomy, and was about to start chemotherapy. She had taken Premarin and Prempro but then switched to bio-identicals after reading *The Sexy Years*. "I really thought hormones were perfectly safe, like when you give insulin to a person with diabetes," she said. "My surgeon said my cancer was invasive and likely caused by hormone replacement. I wish I had never taken it."

As Somers turned out book after book glorifying bio-identicals, the prestigious Mayo Clinic tried to use its famous name to set the record straight. It posted an article on its consumer Web site (www.mayoclinic.com) debunking many of the claims associated with the hormones. And after Winfrey launched her bio-identical push, Lynne Shuster, director of the Women's Health Clinic at Mayo, sent the talk show queen an e-mail imploring her to stop perpetuating the myth that women can take hormones for years on end with no consequences. "I have a problem with the idea of dosing an 80-year-old to achieve outcomes of a 30-year-old," Shuster said. "There's no clinical data supporting its safety. It's excessive. And it's such a contradiction. These people say they're very health oriented. They eat organic foods and exercise regularly. Then they add these supraphysiologic levels of hormones. It's entirely unnatural."

Although anti-aging doctors bragged about their expanding Hollywood clientele, few celebrities other than Somers were bold enough to go public with their hormone regimens. Nick Nolte professed his love for human growth hormone, which he added to his regimen after consulting an anti-aging physician, he explained on *Larry King Live* in February 2000. Nolte was approaching 60 and filming the psychodrama *Affliction* when he discovered HGH. In addition to injecting himself daily, he often carted an IV onto his movie sets so he could infuse himself with high doses of vitamins. At 61, Sylvester Stallone proudly told *Time* magazine that he used testosterone to maintain his youthful stamina and Rocky-esque biceps. "Testosterone to me is so important for a sense of well being when you get older," he said in a January 2008 story. "Everyone over 40 years old would be wise to investigate it because it increases the quality of your life. Mark my words. In 10 years it will be over the counter."

Throughout her three books, Somers unveiled the evolution of her increasingly involved anti-aging routine. She started injecting herself with growth hormone, and she turned her son on to it, too. She took testosterone twice a day, fondly referring to the hormone as "sex in a capsule." Testosterone, she told readers, "does indeed stir things up and make you feel kind of 'wiggly' down there." She then proceeded to lay out a frightening two pages of side effects, including oily skin, deepening voice, and even personality disorders. "People might think you have become aggressive and pushy," she wrote cheerily, seemingly unperturbed by the risks.

Somers said that she bought an infrared sauna so she could "detoxify" herself at home and wore nanotechnology patches at night to help her sleep. The actress launched her own line of cosmetics, which she described in *Breakthrough* as organic and "synthetic free." She interviewed Houston, Texas, anti-aging doctor Steven Hotze, who talked up Armour Thyroid, a thyroid-deficiency treatment that is derived from pig glands. She never explained why she thought pig hormones were healthy but horse hormones were not.

In the introduction to *Breakthrough*, the actress described how she imagined a typical day at age 94. It's the year 2041, she wrote, and she slept soundly and woke up excited and happy. "Most mornings start with wonderful sex with my 105-year-old husband, Alan (who has also embraced the same health regimen)," she wrote. "The two of us are enjoying our lives because along with our healthy, strong bodies, we both have great wisdom and perspective—and this gives us an advantage over younger people." *Breakthrough* raced to the top of the *New York Times* list of best-selling advice books, where it remained for more than 15 weeks.

CHAPTER 6

The Invention of Male Menopause

At the Cenegenics Medical Institute in Las Vegas, patients were made to feel like royalty from the moment they stepped through the front door. To get to the reception desk, they ascended a black and cream marble staircase, framed by majestic columns that made the place look more like an ancient temple than a medical clinic. They spent a full day with doctors, nutritionists, and exercise physiologists, reviewing results from their blood tests and designing diet and workout routines. They got full-body scans to learn whether they had early signs of bone loss or hidden cancers. During breaks, they snacked on PureFit protein bars and Cenegenics private-label springwater while checking their e-mail in private suites overlooking the upscale north Las Vegas neighborhood known as Summerlin. They left with their own tailored menus of hormones, steroids, supplements, and exercise plans. The cost: $3,495, plus tens of thousands more for drugs and follow-up care.

To hear patients Joseph Caprio, Edward Detwiler, and Steven Miller tell it, Cenegenics was the Acropolis of medicine. As much as they cringed at the mention of the M word, they all readily acknowledged that they had come in search of relief from the same sorts of symptoms that menopausal women griped about. "I had lack of energy, fatigue; I put on weight— a lot of weight," said Caprio, 77. Miller, who was 65 and a new-comer to Cenegenics, nodded in agreement. "Sexual drive, emotional drive, being tired—there's a whole variety of things that happen. Whether it's menopausal or not, I don't know. But if you believe age is a disease, there are things you can do to stave it off." Miller hesitated to discuss the specifics of his new Cenegenics regimen, but Caprio and Detwiler were quick to reveal they had used both human growth hormone and testosterone. "I cannot tell you how incredibly great I feel," Detwiler said. "The difference in the stamina, the energy, the focus, the drive, the libido. . . ."

The concept of male menopause, or "andropause," as scien-tists called it, predated the anti-aging industry by about a half-century. But it didn't really catch on until outfits like Cenegenics began courting the aging male.

Although it is true that testosterone levels decline with age, science proved long ago that men didn't suffer anywhere near the sudden hormonal plunges that women did. That made male menopause an inherently incongruous diagnosis—a clin-ical solution to a life passage that previous generations of men sailed right through, without even an inkling that they might need to be "cured." Still, it was a logical progression for an in-dustry in search of a growth path. Anti-aging doctors and phar-macists had already popularized HGH and turned bio-identical hormones into the great antidote against big pharma's supposedly unnatural hot-flash cures. Andropause was the next frontier. And it was conquerable not just with HGH but with the manliest of molecules—testosterone.

Few championed testosterone as vociferously as Alan Mintz, the cofounder of Cenegenics. Mintz, a former radiologist and marathon runner, told *GQ* in 2006 that he started injecting testosterone in his forties and HGH in his fifties. Mintz was working out at 4 a.m. at an all-night gym in Palatine, Illinois, when he met 18-year-old John Adams. Mintz was 25 years older than Adams, but they forged a fast friendship that later blossomed into a business partnership. After Adams graduated from the University of Illinois at Chicago in 1986, he put in a few years as a consultant at Arthur Andersen. Then in 1991, Mintz asked Adams to join him at Medicon, a radiology management company he had founded a few years earlier. They sold Medicon in 1995 for a sum that Adams was not at liberty to reveal, except to say that he and Mintz could have easily retired.

Mintz, then 57, grew more obsessed with healthy living. "We were so into exercise, nutrition, nutraceutical supplementation, vitamins, minerals," Adams recalled. "We would be reading different articles all the time to figure out this supplement or that supplement, and we would actually create our own vitamin packs." Mintz wanted to turn his passion into a business. Instead of waiting for patients to develop symptoms and then scrambling to cure them, Mintz believed he could run them through batteries of tests that would predict their medical vulnerabilities years or even decades in advance. And he could prescribe drugs, food, and exercise to keep people from sliding toward a life of chronic illness. They cofounded Cenegenics in 1997, choosing Las Vegas as the site of their flagship facility because the city lured wealthy retirees. "He was passionate that the paradigm of medicine had to shift," said Adams, who became the company's CEO. Cenegenics quickly went national, and within ten years it housed 45 full-time doctors and 150 "affiliates," who maintained their independent practices but offered the Cenegenics program to patients who wanted to try it. Eighty percent of Cenegenics's patients were men.

Cenegenics's own chief medical officer turned out to be the company's most effective salesman. At age 67, Jeffry Life posed for a print ad, shirtless, revealing bulging abs and pecs that made him look like a 22-year-old pro football player. Life (his real name) smiled broadly, his thumb looped provocatively in a pocket of his low-slung jeans. "You can enjoy youthful aging now!" the ad promised. Life had been injecting HGH and testosterone. Patient Ed Detwiler boasted that Life was his Cenegenics doctor, and the two of them reviewed hormone levels and diet and exercise routines at least twice a year. Detwiler felt sure the shapely physician wouldn't guide him in the wrong direction. It's not "juicing," Detwiler promised, explaining that he wasn't taking superhuman doses of the drugs so much as he was replacing what his body had lost naturally with age. "I have total faith and confidence in Dr. Life," he said.

The notion that men might experience the same change of life that women do was first broadcast by the *Journal of the American Medical Association*, which in 1939 published a piece called "The Male Climacteric." Author August A. Werner, an assistant professor at the St. Louis University School of Medicine, declared, "The condition has probably been overlooked or ignored in men." He wrote at length about a litany of mental and physical symptoms: loss of libido, hot flashes, vertigo, sleeplessness, tingling, crying, memory problems. "The climacteric disturbance may be so severe in some men that they become despondent and develop a psychosis with thoughts of self destruction." Treatment with testosterone, Werner wrote, produced a "remarkable clinical improvement characterized by a marked increase in the erectile capacity and sensitivity of the penis, in the strength of the sex urge and in the capacity to respond with the proper emotions not only to intercourse but also to other acts such as kissing or embracing."

The pharmaceutical industry salivated over the opportunity to forge a new market. Germany-based Schering supplied testosterone to scientists who were studying the hormone's impact on muscle performance in older men. In 1951, the company released a film called *The Male Sex Hormone*, which discussed using testosterone to address male menopause. Despite such ventures, the company failed to generate a frenzy of demand for testosterone. The effort was no doubt hampered by the American Medical Association's outright denunciation of the male climacteric diagnosis.

Then testosterone's reputation became forever tainted by the sports-doping scandals that erupted in the 1990s. Schering's Primobolan was linked to illicit drug use by professional cyclists. And in 1996, Schering bought the German company Jenapharm, which counted among its employees a doctor who had once worked for the legendary East German doping machine. He developed a nasal spray that contained androstenedione, or "andro," the testosterone precursor that would ultimately be banned in sports and added to the list of controlled substances in the United States. As University of Texas at Austin professor John Hoberman wrote in his 2005 book *Testosterone Dreams*, "East German doping expertise was now in the service of a free-market pharmacology looking for mass-market hormone products." Bayer bought Schering in 2006 and continued to market testosterone. But it took the safe route, pushing the product as a treatment for the rare but clinically recognized condition called hypogonadism, which occurs when the testes produce abnormally low levels of testosterone.

It was a much smaller company that finally shoved menopause into the mainstream of male consciousness. In February 2000, Solvay Pharmaceuticals won FDA approval to market AndroGel, a topical form of the steroid. AndroGel was designated to treat hypogonadism, but Solvay took such liberties with its ad campaign that one might think it had found the cure for male malaise. "Fatigued? Depressed Mood? Low Sex Drive?" asked ads the company placed in magazines such as *BusinessWeek*. "Could be your testosterone is running on empty." A gas gauge showing "full" sat next to the drug's logo, with the words "testosterone restored" hovering below. Solvay—a unit of a Belgian conglomerate that until then had been a sleeper in the pharmaceutical world—spent $16 million on TV and print ads from 2002 to 2005, according to market researcher TNS Media Intelligence.

In much the same way that Pfizer had popularized Viagra by coining "erectile dysfunction" and its abbreviation "ED," Solvay hyped "Low T" as a solvable medical problem. The company designed a Web site, Is It Low T? (www.isitlowt.com), where men could learn more about their libido problems and depressed moods. They were invited to "take the Low T quiz," which asked questions like "Have you noticed a decrease in your enjoyment of life?"

Forget hypogonadism. AndroGel had become an all-out escape hatch for middle age. And Solvay's impact on men—their self-image and ultimately their medical decision-making—was eerily reminiscent of the influence Wyeth had had on women with its promotion of Premarin in the mid-20th century. "When anti-aging took off, when we got AndroGel, the male response converged with that of women," said *Testosterone Dreams* author Hoberman. "Once you construct male menopause, you make it obligatory for men to maintain themselves sexually, just like it was obligatory for women."

As AndroGel took off, competitors began devising other convenient ways for men to get their daily testosterone. There was Testim, also a gel, and Striant, a sticky pill that men applied to their upper gums. An upstart called Slate Pharmaceuticals launched Testopel pellets, which emitted testosterone for months after being injected under the skin. Armies of warring salespeople hounded doctors to test patients for low T. Sometimes the competition got nasty. On Cafepharma (www.cafepharma.com), a Web site for pharmaceutical salespeople, an anonymous poster asked how Testim salespeople were competing for AndroGel's market share. A rep replied that he promised that Testim was better absorbed and produced bigger increases in testosterone, and that HMO drug plans were more likely to pay for it. A competitor snapped back, "Oh that Testim stinks something awful! That smell gets into the sheets and clothes and not even hot water and detergent get rid of it."

In February 2009, the Federal Trade Commission (FTC) charged Solvay and two generic drugmakers with conspiring to delay the introduction of generic AndroGel until 2015. The agency alleged that Solvay paid off the generic drugmakers to stop trying to invalidate AndroGel's patents. "At a time of escalating health care costs, these unlawful agreements deny patients the benefit of competition between branded and generic pharmaceuticals and ultimately cost consumers hundreds of millions of dollars a year," an FTC official said in a statement. Solvay said in a statement that its AndroGel patent was valid and that the company intended to use all necessary means to defend the validity of its settlements with the generic drugmakers.

Despite the controversies, Solvay continued to transform AndroGel into a blockbuster. Sales of topical testosterones ballooned from $34 million in 1997 to $750 million in 2008, with AndroGel hauling in nearly three-quarters of the receipts, according to market researcher IMS Health.

The rise of testosterone was enabled by the anti-aging industry's tireless efforts to topple one of the oldest and most widely accepted beliefs about the controversial steroid: that it causes prostate cancer. That danger was first suggested in 1941 by University of Chicago urologist Charles B. Huggins, who published a paper in the journal *Cancer Research* suggesting that prostate cancer "is activated" by testosterone supplementation. Huggins won the Nobel Prize for his work in 1966.

But by the mid-1990s, scientists were starting to question Huggins's methods. Among the doubters was Harvard urologist and associate professor Abraham Morgentaler. In the early 1990s, Morgentaler started performing prostate biopsies on men before he gave them testosterone, just to be safe. Of the first 33 men he tested who had low T, 6 already had prostate cancer. When he presented his findings at a urology meeting in 1996, a colleague in the audience heckled him. "This is garbage," he yelled. "Everyone knows that high T causes prostate cancer, not low T." But Morgentaler kept up his research, and his sleuthing eventually led him to the basement of Harvard Medical School's library, where he found Huggins's original paper. Morgentaler was stunned. Huggins had based his conclusion on a single patient, using a blood test that was intended to show a link between testosterone injections and prostate cancer growth. That test had since been deemed unreliable.

Morgentaler's recounting of his discoveries, the 2008 book *Testosterone for Life*, was instantly canonized by the anti-aging industry. In December 2008, shortly after the book's release, Morgentaler accepted an invitation to speak at A4M's annual conference in Las Vegas. "The idea that testosterone drives cancer is nonsense," the professor said, drawing thunderous applause from the standing-room-only crowd. Morgentaler flipped to a slide that pictured a male lion humping a lioness. "This is a happy guy," joked Morgentaler, a slight man with a high-pitched voice. The next slide showed a lion slumping in a corner, as a nearby female growled at him angrily. "Some of you may recognize this guy."

Then the professor discussed a 61-year-old patient who complained of tiredness, ED, and low libido. His total testosterone was 342 nanograms per deciliter of blood. "Normal" was defined by most mainstream docs as 270–850. Even though the patient wasn't technically a case of low T, Morgentaler treated him with testosterone pellets, which reportedly cured him of his libido problems. As Morgentaler approached the end of his talk, he echoed a refrain that the pioneers of bio-identical hormone replacement used often to validate estrogen therapy for menopausal women: If testosterone were truly dangerous, Morgentaler said, "we should see men in their twenties and thirties with cancer."

Morgentaler's passionate efforts to champion testosterone made him a cause célèbre in the anti-aging world. After his talk, Morgentaler signed copies of *Testosterone for Life* at a booth sponsored by Testopel maker Slate in the A4M trade show. Morgentaler was a paid consultant for the company, and he had received speaking honoraria and other compensation from four other makers of testosterone therapies. But these doctors—the same folks who criticized opponents of bio-identical hormones for being in the pocket of big pharma—greeted Morgentaler as if he were Tom Cruise at a convention of Scientologists. The mob of autograph seekers was so huge Morgentaler could barely move.

Ron Rothenberg of the California Healthspan Institute, the pied piper of HGH, spoke shortly after Morgentaler at A4M. He referred to Morgentaler as his hero, then rattled off references to other research that he said proved high testosterone actually decreased the risk of death. He dismissed reports that testosterone caused men to become mean and unpredictable, behavior commonly known as "roid rage." Speaking quickly—his eyebrows arched as they often were when he was trying to make a point—he looked at the audience and announced, "We're not talking about abuse of anabolic steroids. We're talking about physiologic replacement."

Testosterone was one of the original bio-identicals, synthesized in the 1930s to mimic the real thing. All synthesized testosterones are classified as anabolic steroids, regardless of whether they are FDA approved and for sale at the local pharmacy or passed from a drug dealer to a pro baseball player in the locker room. Anabolic steroids boost appetite, stimulate the bone marrow to make more red blood cells, and promote bone building—attributes that anti-aging doctors said gave testosterone the power to prevent osteoporosis, diabetes, and cardiovascular disease. But testosterone supplements are also androgenic, meaning they control male traits such as the growth of body hair. Too much androgenic firepower can spell trouble: Testosterone lowers sperm count and sometimes causes testicles to shrink. Some men retained water, got pimples, and suffered enlarged prostates or swollen breasts. Others complained of sleep apnea and moodiness.

A few weeks after A4M's show, Morgentaler confessed to feeling conflicted about appearing at an anti-aging conference. "These people are very pro-hormones," he said. "They feel embattled on this particular issue." The spontaneous applause during his presentation caught him off-guard—doctors just don't do that at medical meetings, he said. And he was uncomfortable that anti-aging doctors were so quick to embrace assertions that were not backed up by rigorous scientific support. "I don't consider myself part of the anti-aging crowd," he said. "I'm not sure I'll go to one of their conferences again." Morgentaler was careful to point out that long-term controlled studies of testosterone in healthy aging men—the type of scrutiny that would definitively prove its benefits and risks—had not been done. And he stopped short of recommending the widespread treatment that A4M groupies were promoting.

Despite the anti-aging industry's efforts to distance itself from sports-doping scandals, the two became inevitably linked. Some anti-aging clinics, pharmacies, and Web sites became de facto dealers for pro athletes—and low-hanging fruit for regulators who were looking to stop the spread of banned substances. In 2006, while Operation Phony Pharm and Operation Raw Deal were in full swing, the Albany County District Attorney's Office in New York teamed up with Florida's attorney general and several law enforcement agencies to launch Operation Which Doctor, an effort to shut down steroid trafficking through anti-aging centers. They raided compounders Signature Compounding Pharmacy in Winter Park, Florida, and Applied Pharmacy Services in Mobile, Alabama. At a pharmacy in New York, they seized $7.2 million worth of HGH and a pile of steroid powder imported from China. They charged several doctors with prescribing drugs to pro athletes. Among them was Claire Godfrey, a physician at Infinity Rejuvenation in Deerfield Beach, Florida, who allegedly signed dozens of prescriptions faxed to her by Signature Pharmacy without examining the patients. She pled guilty to one count.

Through it all, anti-aging doctors and their patients defended their testosterone and HGH prescriptions by pointing out that they were only replacing what had been lost with age. They were doing small "physiologic" doses, they said, under strict medical supervision, in contrast to the superhuman doses athletes used.

That substances like testosterone and HGH could be so reviled in sports yet so hallowed in the halls of Cenegenics and its rivals was a testament to the marketing prowess of the anti-aging industry. The industry's promoters took all the signs of normal aging—the beer guts, the limp penises, the foggy memories—and made men believe they were medical problems that could be solved with watered-down versions of dangerous drugs.

As Hoberman put it in *Testosterone Dreams*, "The commercial promotion of various hormone therapies is only one symptom of a profound ethical disorientation within medicine that is gradually changing our sense of what medical science is and what it should be."

Recognizing the potential for abuse, a consortium of five international associations got together in 2008 to publish guidelines for diagnosing and monitoring testosterone deficiency. "Because we saw widespread use of testosterone, and we saw it in older men, we decided we needed to do something," said Christina Wang, director of the Clinical Study Center in Endocrinology, Metabolism, and Nutrition at Harbor-UCLA Medical Center. The guidelines specified that men with testosterone levels of 350 did not need treatment, whereas men whose levels were under 230 did. They suggested that men whose levels fell in between should undergo further testing of both total testosterone and "free testosterone"—that which is available for all the cells of the body to absorb and use.

The gray area between 230 and 350 left a gaping opportunity for anti-aging doctors to focus more on symptoms than on test results. Some rejected the guidelines altogether, recommending that patients boost their testosterone to 500 or even higher if they felt their complaints warranted aggressive treatment. Unreliable testosterone tests further complicated the diagnosis. Glenn Cunningham, a professor at Baylor College of Medicine in Houston, said that a third of men who appeared to have low testosterone when they were tested in the morning turned out to show normal levels later in the day. Testing with different technologies also yielded inconsistent results.

In 2000, a group of scientists led by Cunningham was asked by the National Academies' Institute of Medicine to design a study that would adequately determine the risks and benefits of testosterone replacement in older men. The Cunningham group calculated that they would need to follow 6,000 men for five years in order to detect a 30 percent increase in prostate cancer. But that big a project would have cost $110 million—far more than they could afford because they only had a commitment of $25 million and free testosterone from Solvay. So they had to scale down their plans, settling on a series of smaller studies designed to test the purported benefits of testosterone. In one study, for example, they planned to observe how men receiving testosterone performed on a six-minute walk compared to those getting a placebo. Cunningham hoped the cumulative results might shed some light on the risks of testosterone, too. "But we won't have definitive data for a long time," he warned. The National Institute on Aging set up a testosterone trial in 2009 and began recruiting 800 men at 12 sites around the United States. Results from that trial, however, weren't expected before 2015.

The lack of research caused many members of the medical community to question what testosterone really does in the bodies of aging but otherwise normal men. Ridwan Shabsigh, director of urology at Maimonides Medical Center in New York, believed that the medical literature supported short-term treatment—two years or less—with testosterone, but only in men who underwent regular prostate exams. "We have studies up to a year," Shabsigh said. "To know the exact risk, you need studies that go for 10 to 15 years."

Shabsigh was no prude: In 2007, he published the book *Sensational Sex in 7 Easy Steps: The Proven Plan for Lasting Health and Intimacy*, which encouraged men to have their testosterone levels checked and corrected if necessary. The vivacious professor was a sought-after consultant to companies that made libido-related drugs, including Pfizer, Bayer, and Eli Lilly. But Shabsigh never endorsed the andropause diagnosis, and he worried that the anti-aging industry was using testosterone as a cure for symptoms that could be related to other factors entirely. "Take low mood. Low mood could be part of mild depression," Shabsigh said. "Let's take low energy. Low energy could be related to sleep deprivation, Lyme disease, who knows? Let's take weak muscle power. It could be related simply to lack of exercise. Just being a man and being old and having low testosterone, in my opinion, does not qualify you to have a clinical diagnosis."

The legitimacy of the andropause diagnosis was further muddied when a Finnish study of testosterone in healthy men had to be canceled in 2006. Scientists at the University of Turku in Finland had set out to treat 200 local residents with testosterone and track their results. They sent questionnaires to 30,000 men who were between 40 and 70 years old. Of those who responded, 1,800 reported andropause symptoms. But it turned out that only 250 men actually had low T, and a lot of them were suffering from other diseases. That disqualified them from a study that was designed to look at healthy men. "It's not like we started with a small bunch of people," said the frustrated lead investigator, Antti Perheentupa. "Our finding begs the question, is there such a thing as andropause in men with no diseases, who are living a normal life? Is there any reason to treat healthy men with testosterone at all? The answer is probably no."

Back at Cenegenics, patient Steven Miller turned philosophical on the question of steroids. Miller brought a unique perspective to his anti-aging experience: He had been a pro football player for the Detroit Lions for a few games in 1965, before he was sidelined by a knee injury. Back then, "juicing" meant eating steak and eggs before a game. Athletes didn't lift weights because they were afraid the muscle mass would slow them down, he recalled. Miller had never really thought much about hormones and steroids until he walked into Cenegenics. Just five months into the program, his routine was still evolving, but he was confident that whatever his doctors recommended would be the safe way to go. It would be the right way to go. "What does the data tell you? How do you internalize that?" he pondered. "The only proof you have is the outcome of the blood tests, which are definitive and absolute, and how you feel."

Testosterone therapy had plenty of fans, but those following that type of regimen may have included men who wrecked their marriages, endangered their health, or flat-out lost their minds to hormones and steroids. Angela Pollard, whose name has been changed at her request, was stunned one day in 2005 when her 72-year-old husband announced he was leaving her after 34 years of marriage. He had been injecting himself with HGH and testosterone, which he ordered over the Internet, for the preceding six years. "He said, 'If I weren't doing this, I'd have a pot belly and no sex drive,'" Pollard recalled. He spent more than $1,000 a month on the drugs, then laid down $14,000 for a facelift and $2,000 for Botox injections. He thought he was so healthy that he could stop taking medicine to treat his cardiomyopathy, a dangerous heart condition. That stunt landed him in the hospital, Pollard said. Eventually he moved to the tropics and started dating younger women. "This was pretty childish behavior for a senior citizen."

As testosterone creams and gels became more popular, they started causing bizarre and very scary problems. In 1999, the journal *Pediatrics* published a report of a two-year-old boy who developed pubic hair, acne, and an unusually large penis. Testosterone cream had rubbed off on him from his father, who had been using it on his arm and back. There were other reports of women who developed "hyperandrogenism"—increased body hair, deepening voices, and other male characteristics—when they unknowingly absorbed remnants of testosterone gel used by their husbands or boyfriends. And a 2005 edition of the *European Journal of Pediatrics* published reports on three men who were using testosterone gel for anti-aging purposes. Their daughters had abnormally large bones and clitorises that were far too developed, considering they were under three years old.

On May 7, 2009, the FDA acknowledged the reports of side effects and announced that harsh warning labels would be added to the labels for Solvay's AndroGel and Auxilium Pharmaceuticals' Testim. Diane Murphy, the agency's director of pediatric therapeutics, said the FDA had received at least 20 reports of testosterone exposure in children that resulted in inappropriate genitalia growth, increased libido, aggressive behavior, and other traits that belied their age. During a press conference, she said the agency was concerned about the unapproved testosterone products that were being heavily marketed on the Internet, as well as the rapidly growing off-label use of testosterone gel by women, who were embracing it as the female Viagra. The FDA estimated that about 25,000 of the 1.4 million prescriptions written for AndroGel in 2007 were doled out to women. Solvay and Auxilium were instructed to add warnings about "secondary exposure" and specific instructions for minimizing the risk, including this warning: "Adults should wash the application site thoroughly with soap and warm water prior to any situation where skin-to-skin contact with another person is anticipated."

Cenegenics CEO John Adams went to great lengths to prove his doctors were properly trained to prescribe hazardous substances. He set up a not-for-profit education and research foundation, which put new doctor recruits through five days of intensive training, plus additional hours of home study. All his physicians completed "mini-residencies," which involved spending three days with a Cenegenics veteran, before they could strike out on their own. Still, Cenegenics's program didn't remotely match the training that true hormone specialists go through. Endocrinologists who were certified by the American Board of Medical Specialties endured two years of rigorous training, including a full year in a clinical setting. Only two board-certified endocrinologists joined Cenegenics in its first decade.

Patients were untroubled by this. By 2008, Cenegenics had 15,000 patients and was pulling in $50 million a year. At the annual conference of A4M's competitor, the Age Management Medicine Group (AMMG), held at a swank resort in Boca Raton, Florida, in 2009, Adams told an audience of 200 doctors that his company had barely cracked the market. "We believe there are 14 million people who can afford our program," he said. He went on to promise that any doctor who joined the company could expect to bring home as much as $350,000 a year, for just 55 hours of work per week.

The Cenegenics success inspired other entrepreneurs to franchise the anti-aging concept. In 2003, identical-twin brothers Paul and Patrick Savage founded BodyLogicMD and turned it into the McDonald's of medicine. Paul was an emergency room doctor in Chicago, and Patrick was a marketing executive in Jacksonville, Florida. "I was 267 pounds and I didn't feel well," Paul recalled. "I was worn down, stressed out." An anti-aging doctor put him on DHEA and growth hormone, and he started eating better and exercising. The brothers hadn't seen each other in years, so Paul decided to spend Christmas in Florida. By then, his weight had fallen to 180, and he was ripped and full of energy. Patrick, on the other hand, was 280 pounds, out of shape, and struggling to control his cholesterol. Paul recalled that his brother opened the door and uttered a single stunned word: "Wow." Then, said Paul, Patrick's wife came to the door, "and she was like, 'Oh wow, oh wow.'"

Paul wanted to leave the ER and start his own anti-aging office in Chicago, so he asked his brother to help him manage the business side of the practice. When they decided to expand, Patrick tackled the venture as if he were designing a whole new medical system. At first, he and Paul signed on as a Cenegenics affiliate, and both went through the company's $3,500 new-patient assessment so they could better understand how the incumbent treated its patients. Patrick deemed Cenegenics a bit over-the-top. "In that initial eight-hour session, I got one hour with a doctor, two hours with a nutritionist, and three hours in a spa getting a massage," Patrick recalled. He figured BodyLogic could cut out the spa services and offer anti-aging medicine for a fraction of the price.

BodyLogic attracted prospective patients through the Internet and got bulk-purchasing deals on everything from blood testing to brochures. "What one physician can't afford, many can when they band together," Paul reasoned. Patrick soon joined the anti-aging club, starting a regimen of hormones and supplements, monitored by Paul.

Initially, BodyLogic operated like a consultancy. Doctors who joined the network managed their own practices and paid fees to the parent company for marketing and technology support. But the physicians were overwhelmed by clerical work, so Patrick shifted to more of a traditional franchise model. He hired 25 people to find prospective patients, order up their blood and saliva tests, and schedule their appointments with BodyLogic doctors. The twins' three sisters soon joined the company to help out with marketing and administrative tasks. Doctors paid franchise fees when they first started up, but BodyLogic augmented those revenues with pharmacy and lab-testing receipts. Cenegenics also made most of its sales from lab and pharmacy services, Adams told doctors at AMMG's Boca Raton convention.

Within a few short years, BodyLogic had recruited 25 doctors in 14 states. Its patient base was growing by 35 percent a year. But most of the patients were women, so in 2008, BodyLogic turned its attention to andropause. A June 2008 press release declared, "Hot Flash Husbands and Hormonal Dads for Father's Day: BodyLogicMD Helps Men Understand Andropause for National Men's Health Week." Chief Medical Officer Alicia Stanton was quoted in the release declaring that once men hit their thirties, they begin losing testosterone at a rate of 1 to 2 percent per year. "It can take more than a decade for symptoms of andropause to appear, but men need to realize that it isn't just a matter of aging," she said. The release referred vaguely to experts who purportedly estimated that 25 million American men over age 40 were suffering from andropause.

Despite the lack of rigorous science behind the campaign, it was oddly effective. By the end of 2008, almost 30 percent of BodyLogic's patients were men. Stanton in particular saw a flood of new male patients at her Connecticut clinic. Bruce Whipple, 55, was sold after just a few months of trying testosterone cream, bio-identical progesterone, DHEA, and a cocktail of other remedies Stanton prescribed. Whipple was a marketing exec for RBC Bearings and an active marathoner and biker. But he couldn't sleep, and he was often famished in the middle of the night. The hormones and steroids, which he estimated would run him $3,000 a year, got his sleep and his weight back on track, he said, enough so that he was planning a 100-mile bike ride. "I always said I'd live to 120," he said. "I want to be in condition to continue to run, cycle, and swim." During a follow-up appointment, he told Stanton about a nutritionist he had started consulting. "She asked if you were an endocrinologist," Whipple said to Stanton. The doctor replied, "I am in a way, but I'm not board certified."

By the mid-2000s, anti-aging pioneers were finding new ways to capitalize on the male menopause concept. BodyLogic added a symptom to its andropause menu called "irritable male syndrome (IMS)." The IMS link on the company's Web site pointed to a page headlined, "Look out! He's gonna blow!" IMS, it explained, strikes men between the ages of 40 and 60 and is marked by anger, sarcasm, frustration, impatience, and even hostility. The cause, the company said, was an imbalance of hormones, in particular testosterone.

Irritable male syndrome was first popularized by Jed Diamond, a psychotherapist in northern California, who announced the new malady in a 2004 book called *The Irritable Male Syndrome*. Diamond, an andropause specialist, had been corresponding with men via his Web site, MenAlive.com (www.menalive.com), and he had become fascinated by reports of personality changes in midlife. "I found a set of symptoms tied to irritability and anger," he said. "A lot of men had these issues." Women were e-mailing him, as well. "They were saying, 'I'm walking on eggshells around my husband. I don't know if he'll be nice or mean.'" Diamond was going to call the phenomenon "Jekyll and Hyde Syndrome," but then he happened upon the work of a British scientist named Gerald Lincoln, who had already coined the term "irritable male syndrome." Lincoln, a senior research fellow at the University of Edinburgh Medical School, had announced the new ailment a few years earlier in a paper published in the journal *Reproduction, Fertility, and Development.*

Lincoln spent much of his career studying the behavior and physiology of the Soay ram, a black, horned creature whose testosterone levels fall naturally at the end of each mating season. At that time, the animals become agitated and short-tempered, fighting so viciously with other males that they end up covered in gashes. In the paper, Lincoln defined IMS as "a behavioural state of nervousness, irritability, lethargy, depression and low libido that occurs in adult male mammals following withdrawal of T."

Granted, humans don't suffer seasonal declines in testosterone, Lincoln admitted. But subsequent studies on men who were asked to document their symptoms after withdrawing from testosterone convinced Lincoln that human males weren't all that different from Soay sheep. "Many aspects of their mood were affected," Lincoln said. "They were tense, irritable, and they recorded this in their diaries."

After Diamond published his book on IMS, he garnered further enthusiasm for the new ailment by developing the Irritable Male Syndrome Program. For $39, men could go online to correspond with other IMS sufferers and get coached on various methods for dealing with hormone imbalances. In 2004, Diamond produced *The Male Menopause Workshop*, a PBS series that ran during pledge week in Chicago. And in October 2008, he was featured on CBS's *Early Show* as part of a series the program titled "Men Behaving Badly." Diamond explained to correspondent Julie Chen that there were nine common species of IMS-stricken men, including "Grumpy," "Fearful," and "Unappreciated." He revealed that all three of the show's male stars—Harry Smith, Russ Mitchell, and Dave Price—tested positive on the IMS quiz. Without pointing fingers, he said slyly that one was "Grumpy," another was "Exhausted," and the third was "Impulsive."

Back in Scotland, Lincoln was bemused and a little annoyed. He had never intended to imply that all men might suffer hormonal changes, nor did he believe they all needed testosterone therapy. "At what point do you recommend testosterone supplementation?" he asked. "It's very complicated. There are negative effects." The invention of andropause, he added, left men with the same predicament facing women: Anti-aging proponents were telling them that hormones and steroids were natural, yet there was no scientific proof that taking them throughout their golden years was a good idea. "At the end of the day," Lincoln asked, "when do you stop?"

In April 2009, TV psychologist Dr. Phil joined the pro-hormone chorus, airing a show that included a discussion of male menopause. Dr. Phil's wife, Robin McGraw, repeated the story she had told on *Oprah* and again featured the California anti-aging center run by Prudence Hall. A patient named Howard was shown consulting with one of Hall's physicians. "When I look in the mirror, I don't see an attractive man. I see a man who's full of failure and doubt," Howard said. His testosterone level was 347—well above what endocrinologists would classify as low T. But the doctor recommended boosting him to 550. "I'll do 800 if you want," Howard said. Just 36 hours later, the patient reported he was a new man. "Brain feels a lot sharper," he said. "I feel a lot stronger now than I used to feel."

Traffic to BodyLogic's Web site had jumped 225 percent after Winfrey's shows on menopause and bio-identical hormones, forcing the company to install two extra servers and quadruple its phone capacity. Web interest jumped another 10 percent after Dr. Phil's endorsement, and BodyLogic's revenues were growing 150 percent a year.

Paul Savage had left BodyLogic the previous year, choosing to focus on patient care and research rather than on building the franchise that had become his brother's obsession. Patrick remained a staunch believer, unapologetic and undaunted. "With all due respect, I was in banking and it seemed to me that people there made some choices that really weren't all that smart," said Patrick, who had worked for AT&T Universal Card and Tyco prior to founding BodyLogic. "It's not that different from this industry. There are aspects of this that even I don't agree with. But as a whole do I think we're helping people make educated life choices about their health? Absolutely."

Patrick had testosterone pellets implanted under the skin of his rear hip, which helped him correct what he believed to be "suboptimal" levels of the steroid. He was aware of the FDA-approved product Testopel, but he chose to use testosterone pellets made by a BodyLogic compounding pharmacy instead. "Problem is, Testopel is 75 milligrams, so I'd have to insert so many of them," Patrick said. "They're able to be compounded in a larger size. We find that to be more effective." Savage didn't worry that the compounded drugs BodyLogic encouraged patients to buy were untested in large, rigorous trials. "We don't have a lot of long-term double-blind studies on most stuff," he pointed out. "With all due respect, I don't believe it would matter that much from a marketing standpoint."

In 2009, Cenegenics's poster boy Jeffry Life posed for a new set of ads at the age of 70, dressed in a sleeveless muscle shirt. Life had recently left his position as Cenegenics's chief medical officer, but he continued to practice with the company as an affiliate and remained convinced that testosterone was safe to prescribe to his patients. Life was fond of telling the story of having once looked up the words "aging" and "disease" in *Dorland's Medical Dictionary* and discovering that aging was not defined as a disease, but hormone loss was. "When we see patients with declining IGF-1 levels, low testosterone, it's our responsibility to do something about it," said Life at the Age Management Medicine Group's Boca Raton conference. "I believe aging is a disease. We need to cure it. If we don't, we're violating our oath." Life was the star presenter at the conference, and he cheerfully told the attendees that he had been injecting testosterone twice a day for six years.

During a quiet break from the event, Life reflected on the controversies surrounding testosterone replacement. "According to the recent scientific evidence, testosterone supplementation in clinically deficient men is without problems as long as levels are monitored routinely and values do not become superphysiologic," he said. "If I hadn't treated my clinically proven testosterone deficiency with testosterone supplementation, I would not only have been forced to retire years ago, but very well might have died due to complications from full-blown cardio-metabolic syndrome."

However, for Cenegenics's godfather of testosterone, Alan Mintz, steroids were clearly not the key to eternal youth. In June 2007, at the age of 69, Mintz died while undergoing a brain biopsy. Cenegenics's CEO Adams said Mintz had noticed some memory issues and had been hoping that a biopsy would help diagnose the problem.

But anti-aging critics weren't buying Cenegenics's story. After all, it's unlikely any surgeon would recommend as drastic a procedure as a brain biopsy for someone in his sixties who was getting a little forgetful. Boston University professor Perls posted the news of Mintz's passing on his Web site Growth Hormone/HGH/Antiaging and Sports under the heading "Anti-aging docs dying young." Perls had seen a newspaper article saying that Mintz suffered an accident in the gym, so he sent it to the coroner's office in Las Vegas with a note asking why they didn't investigate the accident. "They didn't think there was any foul play. That's all they cared about," Perls said. "If you look at the literature of why a neurosurgeon would do a biopsy, 99.9% of the time it's because there's some mass. Either you worry about the mass being some kind of infection that you can treat, or it's a brain tumor, or it's benign. [Cenegenics] did an unbelievable job of burying it." In response to this claim, Adams said Cenegenics did not understand Perls's accusation and thought it was irresponsible.

In 2006, Mintz had declared anti-aging drugs to be safe during a segment broadcast on *60 Minutes*. Correspondent Steve Kroft commented that there were no controlled studies proving that the types of treatment regimens Cenegenics prescribed—and that Mintz himself was taking—actually relieved the frailties of old age. Mintz, clearly bothered, replied, "We've never done a double-blind study on the sun, but you know and I

know even on a cloudy day it's coming up every morning."
Kroft asked Mintz if he was sure the treatments wouldn't ultimately prove to be detrimental 5, 10, or even 15 years down
the line. "If you talk about 5, 10, 15 years," Mintz answered,
"I'm pretty comfortable." One year later, Mintz was dead.

CHAPTER 7

Ragtag Pharmacists Cash In

On February 26, 2007, Signature Compounding Pharmacy owners Stan and Naomi Loomis were indicted as part of Operation Which Doctor, the joint effort between Florida and New York to clamp down on illegal steroid trafficking. Albany County district attorney P. David Soares released a two-page statement laying out a dramatic list of criminal acts allegedly committed by the Florida pharmacists. They filled bogus prescriptions from New York physicians, Soares said, and sold testosterone, nandrolone, and other controlled substances. Stan Loomis's brother, Mike Loomis, who was head pharmacist, and pharmacy employees Kirk Calvert and Tony Palladino were also named in the indictment. A picture of the pharmacy's headquarters was posted prominently on Soares's Web site, along with headshots of the Loomises and Calvert, surrounded by eight anti-aging centers. Red lines connected Signature to boxed photos of each of the anti-aging clinics, as if to imply that the pharmacy was the headquarters of a dangerous crime ring.

Among the doctors pictured there was Claire Godfrey, the Infinity Rejuvenation physician who had been indicted along with Signature.

It was a stunning turn of events for Signature, which was known in the anti-aging world as a leading supplier of specially tailored, "natural" menopause and andropause hormones. Prosecutors estimated that the pharmacists grossed about $30 million in 2006. And the *Orlando Sentinel* reported that the Loomises were building a $6 million home to add to their collection of real estate, which also included a $1.8 million, 6,000-square-foot mansion in Isleworth, an Orlando country club. Now they were facing up to 25 years in prison.

The five Signature employees pled not guilty, and less than two years later, an Albany judge threw out the indictment. The judge, Stephen W. Herrick, blamed the prosecutors for frequently changing the counts against Signature, causing grand jury members to become confused. "The grand jury was not advised as to which counts charged which particular crimes and, apparently were left to sift through the voluminous amount of materials and exhibits introduced," Herrick wrote in the September 2008 decision. A stupid mistake, in other words— but one serious enough to knock the wind right out of Operation Which Doctor.

Pharmaceutical compounding seemed to be a shadow industry. Compounders assembled their own drug recipes in back rooms of neighborhood apothecaries or bare-bones manufacturing shops they built themselves. As the anti-aging industry created a market for bio-identical hormones and other alternative treatments, compounders found themselves increasingly in demand. But they were almost completely unsupervised by any regulatory body. Federal laws meant to protect consumers from dangerous drugs were so convoluted that compounders could easily skirt around them. State pharmacy boards, which were supposed to police drugstores, rarely had enough manpower to monitor every compounder. The more popular compounded drugs became, the further pharmacists dug themselves into politicians' pockets, making hundreds of thousands of dollars of contributions to the legislators who were most likely to preserve their freedom to compound. And if it were not for the sports-doping scandals that erupted in the late 1990s, compounding pharmacies probably wouldn't have ever had to worry about getting in trouble.

Compounders were the original drugmakers, preparing custom doses of therapeutic brews and salves at the dawn of modern medicine. In the 1930s, more than half of all prescriptions were compounded. But then industrial manufacturing took over, big pharma was born, and the demand for pharmacy-made preparations plummeted. For much of the middle part of the 20th century, compounding was a niche trade, practiced by a select group of pharmacists who would fill prescriptions for tailored medicines. A compounder might put a pain drug into a lollipop for a child with cancer, for example, or turn a pill into syrup for an elderly patient who had trouble swallowing. In compounding, this arrangement was known as the "triad"—one pharmacist filling one doctor's prescription for one patient. It was not lucrative, but it was perfectly legal and useful.

Just as the anti-aging industry was on the rise, President Bill Clinton signed a law that inadvertently allowed compounders to bust out of the triad. The Food and Drug Administration Modernization Act of 1997 (FDAMA) exempted compounders from having to seek approval to market their homemade drugs and from having to abide by the strict manufacturing practices that big pharma followed. Their only obligation was to follow a few simple rules. They had to use ingredients from already-approved drugs, for example, and they couldn't advertise their compounded products. Suddenly a cloud lifted: Pharmacists no longer had to worry about the FDA busting down their doors and demanding they register their products or manufacture them using strict quality-control measures.

FDAMA also allowed pharmacists to cut free from managed care, which was so squeezing their drug reimbursements that they had to look elsewhere for profits. Anti-aging and compounding were a match born of financial opportunism: Patients were willing to pay cash for hormone mixtures that their doctors said they couldn't get from drug companies, and pharmacists were more than happy to fill the demand.

Pharmacist Eric Fox was a case in point. He owned a neighborhood shop in Berwyn, Pennsylvania, that filled traditional prescriptions and billed them to insurance companies. In 2004, he decided to split off a second shop, Compounding Rx Apothecary, which was almost entirely cash based. That store flourished, while his original shop slowly went bust. "My insurance reimbursements fell drastically," said Fox. "I'd pay $200 for a drug and get reimbursed $205. It wasn't enough for me to keep that shop open."

So Fox went into compounding full-time, settling in a Malvern, Pennsylvania, strip mall, a few doors down from a pizza shop and a doggie day care center. Compounding Rx Apothecary looked like a throwback to the 19th century. A large sign in the window advertised New Emu Pain Relief, a cream made from the giant bird's feather oil. The sign urged customers to use it to treat the pain from arthritis, sciatica, carpal tunnel syndrome, shingles, leg cramps, fibromyalgia, and neuropathy, as well as neck, back, and knee pain. Inside, the handprints of the anti-aging industry were everywhere. Fox was dressed in a white lab coat, mixing up drug medleys behind the pharmacy counter. Brochures near his cash register advertised compounded testosterone for andropause therapy and bio-identical hormones for menopause. "I get calls all the time from people asking me to speak to their doctors about hormone-replacement therapy," Fox said. "There's a lot of interest." He never missed the old days of submitting claims to tightfisted managed-care companies. "This is better economically," he said.

Brothers Joe and John Grasela were also driven out of mainstream pharmacy practice. They owned ten pharmacies in San Diego until managed care sopped up all their profits. In 1993, they opened University Compounding Pharmacy and established themselves as anti-aging pioneers, teaming up with A4M and high-profile physicians such as Ron Rothenberg to spread the hormone gospel. "Hormones became the driving force," said John Grasela during a break from the 2006 training conference he and his brother put on with Rothenberg. "There was more and more demand, and we just ran with it." By the mid-2000s, hormones accounted for 75 percent of University's sales. And Grasela himself had joined the anti-aging bandwagon, ingesting many of the supplements and hormones he was promoting. "I'm in the best shape of my whole life," said Grasela, then 57. "I'm leaner, I have more energy, my thinking process is better." To maintain his muscular physique, he only had to work out for 15 minutes three times a week, he said. "I get more bang for my buck. The hormones are helping."

Regardless of whether compounding pharmacists were shooting up HGH or slathering on testosterone cream, they were all clearly committed to the anti-aging credo. They seemed to dismiss the idea that the drugs they sold (and often took themselves) might be dangerous. And they repeated the same claims that anti-aging doctors used to recruit patients. "If hormones were dangerous, why don't young people have heart attacks and cancer?" Grasela asked. "This is what the body makes. We're only giving the amounts that are needed to get back to normal levels."

Fox, the Graselas, and others found like-minded pharmacists in the Professional Compounding Centers of America (PCCA), an organization founded in 1981 when a Houston pharmacist was asked to compound an antinausea medication that was no longer on the market. The pharmacist started networking with other compounders and eventually figured out how to find the chemicals he needed to make the drug. Those compounders built PCCA as the go-to supplier for software, education, and—most importantly—chemicals. As the anti-aging industry took hold, PCCA's membership rolls ballooned, from a handful of pharmacists to 3,500.

Ten years after the launch of PCCA, the International Academy of Compounding Pharmacists (IACP) emerged in suburban Houston. It promoted itself as an independent organization that "fought to protect, promote and advance the art and science of the compounding pharmacy profession." But its ties to the chemical industry were evident from the start, and not just because of its close proximity to PCCA. David Sparks, who was CEO of PCCA, was also a founding director of IACP. And IACP received contributions from other companies that sold chemicals to compounders, such as Gallipot of St. Paul, Minnesota.

Free of FDA oversight, some compounders began mixing up giant batches of hormones—far more than what a single doctor would need for a single patient—and keeping the extra on hand in case other customers might want to try the mixtures. Despite FDAMA's restrictions on advertising, some started hawking homemade brews with names like Natural Radiance Estriol Creme and Natural Woman Progesterone Cream on the Internet. Neighborhood pharmacists led seminars on hormone replacement and appeared as menopause experts on local TV and radio shows.

During a November 2005 radio talk show, compounder Stan Scarbrough of Findlay, Ohio, urged women to come to his pharmacy and pick up questionnaires to fill out at home about their health. Scarbrough told the show's host that he would read each questionnaire and meet with the patient for 45 minutes. Then he would put together a suggested formula of hormones. "We send physicians our recommendations," Scarbrough said. "Quite frankly, the dosage we start a patient on is an educated guess," he added jovially. "I have some patients that call me 'doctor' by accident." Listeners may not have realized that in 2001, the Ohio State Board of Pharmacy charged Scarbrough with selling several adulterated or misbranded drugs and put him on probation for five years. Some of the samples the board uncovered were hormones that lacked expiration dates.

As compounders became more and more visible, consumer-protection watchdogs began to speak up. One vocal critic was Gregg Jones, a pharmacy inspector for the Florida Department of Health. Pharmacists in his state weren't just compounding anti-aging hormones. They were also making copies of popular drugs to treat respiratory ailments such as asthma. The pharmacists discovered that they could earn more money by mixing up the respiratory drugs themselves—using ingredients they bought at dirt-cheap bulk rates from PCCA and other sources—and then billing Medicare as if they were selling the FDA-approved versions.

Jones began showing up at compounding pharmacies unannounced, documenting his discoveries of careless and less-than-sterile manufacturing practices. At one pharmacy, Jones watched a woman in the mail room fill vials of respiratory medications and then cap each one with her ungloved hands. At another drugstore, which was making a medicine to treat impotence—the designated compounding area looked like the pharmacy version of a teenager's bedroom: Vials and syringes were strewn across a table, and ingredients were arranged haphazardly on shelves and in boxes. One pharmacy owner commented to an inspector that making an injectable drug was like baking a cake. "You just do the math and mix." As Jones traveled from pharmacy to pharmacy, he was appalled to find ingredients stored in bathrooms, or in refrigerators, right next to the pharmacists' lunches.

On July 14, 2000, Jones presented some of his discoveries to an FDA advisory committee. Panel member and physician Elizabeth McBurney asked him to estimate how many of the hundreds of pharmacies that were compounding in Florida were doing so properly. "Most of the smaller pharmacies," Jones replied, "are not following any type of controls in producing [drugs]."

And Florida wasn't the only place where sloppy compounding was putting patients at risk. In 2001, six customers of Physicians Pharmacy in Austell, Georgia, received compounded thyroid medications that were hundreds of times more potent than what their doctors had prescribed. Three ended up in the hospital. The owner of the pharmacy, John Marzullo, surrendered his license. The following year, four patients contracted meningitis from an injectable pain drug that Urgent Care Pharmacy in Spartanburg, South Carolina, had prepared and sent to clinics in several states. One patient died. And in 2003, Portage Pharmacy in Portage, Michigan, had to recall 791 vials of compounded drugs that had become contaminated.

In Missouri, it took a crime of monstrous proportions to spark a major overhaul of the compounding laws. Kansas City pharmacist Robert R. Courtney pled guilty in 2002 to diluting chemotherapy drugs, which he admitted may have affected 4,200 cancer patients. He was sentenced to 30 years in prison. State regulators were already considering tightening up controls on compounders. But the Courtney arrest "sped things up," recalled the Missouri Board of Pharmacy's then executive director Kevin Kinkade. "The need to update the rules took center stage." The board rewrote standards for sterility and required more detailed labeling on compounded products. The state upped the pharmacy board's budget by 35 percent and set aside funding to add two inspectors. Board employees began making undercover drug buys from compounders, either in person or via the Web, so the state could monitor compounded products for sterility and potency.

Between 2003 and 2005, Missouri collected and tested 410 products. More than 15 percent of the drugs were not as potent as the pharmacists claimed they were, and a few contained no active ingredients at all. All together, 81 samples collected from 59 pharmacies tested outside the acceptable limits for potency—a failure rate of 20 percent. About a third of the unacceptable products were made of estrogen, progesterone, or testosterone. Regulators shared the results with the pharmacists in the hopes that shining a light on the problems would be enough to improve the quality of compounded products.

They were wrong. In the year ended June 2007, 24 percent of samples collected from Missouri pharmacies failed potency tests. Ten of the 51 failures were menopause hormones.

The effort to expose the dangers of compounded drugs soon went national. In its August 2006 edition of the newsletter *Worst Pills, Best Pills News,* consumer watchdog Public Citizen shouted, "DO NOT USE Bio-identical Hormone Replacement Therapy (BHRT) Manufactured by Compounding Pharmacists." Larry Sasich, a pharmacist, wrote the article as a counterpoint to the compounders' propaganda. "Proponents of BHRT, those benefiting economically from their sale, maintain that the right of women and their doctors to choose must be protected," Sasich wrote. "This is a perversion of consumerism often put forward by producers of shoddy products. There is a more fundamental right that is being violated by compounding pharmacies: the right to a marketplace free of potentially dangerous untested products promoted for unsubstantiated uses."

Sasich worked at Public Citizen in Washington, D.C., for ten years, and when FDAMA was passed, he became one of its most vocal critics. "I thought it could be used to make an end run around the drug-approval process," he said. During the 2000 FDA hearing, Sasich spoke just after Florida's Jones showed his slides of subpar compounding conditions. Sasich said, "I think one of the issues that this committee has to think about is, there is no longer any effective regulatory route for preventing or protecting the public from these kinds of activities. That was eliminated with FDAMA."

Sasich was often surprised by how openly some pharmacists violated FDA restrictions. It may have been tempting for them to flaunt rules about using FDA-approved ingredients because they knew that the FDA had limited resources to monitor them. As an experiment, Sasich once called a compounder in The Plains, Virginia, and asked if he would fill two prescriptions for drugs made of cyclandelate and piracetam, substances that some doctors thought could improve blood flow and cognition. The drugs were not on the market in the United States, and when Sasich told the pharmacist that the prescribing physician was licensed in Washington, D.C., "he said, 'I don't care if he's licensed in Bosnia, I'll fill these.'"

Unapproved ingredients were ridiculously easy for compounders to find. The PCCA's 2006 catalog offered cyclandelate ($35 for 25 grams) and piracetam ($17 for 25 grams). The 300-page tome was also a source of domperidone, a drug that was prescribed in some countries to induce lactation and relieve nausea. FDA officials had issued a public warning about domperidone two years earlier because they had seen published reports of patients suffering arrhythmias, cardiac arrest, and sudden death. The agency also sent six warning letters to pharmacies caught compounding the substance.

Other advocacy organizations piled into the grassroots effort to control compounding. In the 1990s, a Fairfax, Virginia, group called Allergy and Asthma Network Mothers of Asthmatics (AANMA) began collecting samples of copycat asthma drugs that they believed were being compounded illegally. Founder Nancy Sander had spent years struggling to manage her daughter's asthma, and she was disturbed to discover how prevalent shoddily compounded inhalers had become. So she and the other mothers in her group began documenting cases of patients who were sickened by compounded respiratory drugs. Then they started knocking on senators' doors. Sander explained to them that PCCA and IACP—contrary to their public personas as the protectors of community pharmacies—were really just conduits for chemical companies that wanted to support their growing market of compounders. "It's a sham," said Sander. "It's a shell game."

The rapidly growing influence of compounders over physicians hit a little too close to home for Sander. When she was 55, she consulted her doctor for help dealing with menopause. The doctor urged her to take a saliva test and told her she should buy compounded hormones from a pharmacy in Virginia. Her doctor didn't bother to tell her there were FDA-approved alternatives to Premarin and Prempro. Sander was mortified that her own physician was blind to the risks of compounding. "She only talked about how dangerous prescription drugs were," Sander said. "She didn't discuss the options."

When it came to controlling the rapidly growing compounding industry, the FDA was caught in a legal quagmire. Its troubles began in 2001 with a ruling in the U.S. Court of Appeals for the Ninth Circuit, encompassing nine western states. In the case, *Thompson v. Western States Medical Center*, a group of pharmacists challenged the advertising restrictions in FDAMA, saying that they violated their First Amendment rights to commercial free speech. The court agreed. But the part of FDAMA that described the advertising limit, section 503A, also laid out all the other restrictions for compounders, including the requirement that they only compound with ingredients from FDA-approved drugs. The court ruled, however, that the marketing restrictions could not be separated from the other parts of section 503A. Effectively, then, they struck down the entire compounding section of FDAMA as unconstitutional.

The case went all the way to the U.S. Supreme Court, which upheld the pharmacists' right to commercial free speech in a 2002 ruling.

But the Supreme Court justices left a lot of unanswered questions. Should compounded drugs be considered "new" drugs? Should pharmacists have to abide by the rest of section 503A, even though they had regained their right to advertise? The justices didn't say. So the FDA decided to take the lead, reissuing a ten-year-old "compliance policy guide" on compounding. That guide laid out boundaries for compounding pharmacists. For example, the agency said it could take enforcement action against a pharmacy using bulk ingredients that were not components of FDA-approved drugs. It could also crack down on pharmacists who were compounding drugs that had been taken off the market for safety reasons or who were making bulk quantities in anticipation of receiving prescriptions.

An all-out war broke out between the FDA and the pharmacists. The agency continued to send warning letters to pharmacists, invoking its rights to take action under the compliance policy guide. Pharmacists answered by insisting that the Supreme Court had invalidated the guide and more or less emasculated the FDA on all matters of compounding.

In September 2004, one anti-aging doctor decided to try to resolve the issue in court once and for all. Steven Hotze, a former ER doctor who owned the Hotze Health and Wellness Center and compounding pharmacy in suburban Houston, formed a coalition of ten pharmacies and sued the FDA. Hotze was riding a wave of public support for anti-aging medicine. A few months earlier, he had testified in favor of bio-identicals before Congress—dismissing critic Adriane Fugh-Berman by suggesting that she get worked up at his clinic. He often appeared on

Texas TV news programs, preaching the value of bio-identical hormones to treat everything from panic attacks to migraines to memory loss. The pharmacists, who came to be known as the Midland Coalition, alleged that the FDA was illegally enforcing a regulation that it never had the authority to issue. "The FDA's unlawful actions are meant to intimidate law-abiding pharmacists to quit compounding medications," Hotze said in a press release.

The Midland Coalition included some of the anti-aging industry's VIPs. There was Graselas's University Compounding Pharmacy, plus College Pharmacy in Colorado Springs, Colorado, and Applied Pharmacy Services in Mobile. The pharmacists set up a legal defense fund, and within a few short weeks, they had raised more than half of the $1.5 million they projected they would need to fight the case. Hotze was a magnet for anti-aging advocates, easily garnering support and funding for his pro-compounding fights. And he did it without ever joining A4M or even attending one of its conferences, he said. "I'm not a big joiner. I'm just not," claimed Hotze, a native Texan with a propensity to ramble. "I don't need to be part of anything to get value. I'm kinda like a maverick. I'm a free enterprise guy."

A district court judge ruled that compounded drugs were not subject to FDA restrictions—a victory for Hotze and his followers. But the FDA appealed, and in July 2008, the U.S. Court of Appeals for the Fifth Circuit overturned the Midland decision, concluding that compounded products were new drugs and that pharmacists preparing them must abide by everything in 503A except the advertising restrictions. The conflicting court decisions raised questions about whether compounders in some states had more freedom than those in other states. But the FDA continued to enforce its restrictions nationwide.

In an apparent attempt to convince the public that its practices were aboveboard, the compounding industry developed an accreditation program in 2006. The Pharmacy Compounding Accreditation Board (PCAB) incorporated itself in Washington, D.C., and began taking applications from pharmacies that wanted a seal of approval to show they were adhering to standards of quality and sterility. "They want an independent board to come in and set quality standards they can live with," said Kenneth Baker, who was PCAB's first executive director. The organization boasted that there were eight major pharmacy associations on its governing board, including IACP. "We are excited to work with this diverse group of leading pharmacy organizations," said IACP executive director L. D. King in a statement.

But the notion that the PCAB was either diverse or independent was questionable. Half the governing board was made up of organizations that—like the IACP—earned much of their income from dues or other fees paid by pharmacists, drugmakers, and chemical suppliers. It depended on annual fees paid by pharmacists, not to mention contributions from companies that were profiting from compounding. Among the list of PCAB's biggest contributors: chemical suppliers Professional Compounding Centers of America and Spectrum, as well as Labrix Clinical Services, a major seller of the blood and saliva tests anti-aging doctors used to determine which compounded drugs to prescribe to their patients. "PCAB is not recognized by any regulatory body for any purpose," griped Sasich. "It's compounders monitoring compounders."

In July 2007, Midland Coalition member College Pharmacy earned its PCAB accreditation, an accomplishment owner and pharmacist Thomas Bader bragged about prominently on his Web site at the time. "College Pharmacy Joins Elite Few to Earn PCAB Accreditation," the headline blared. "We are honored by this new accreditation," said Bader in a statement on the site. "It confirms our commitment to providing safe, personalized solutions that meet the medical needs of our patients—and the needs of the healthcare providers in our community who rely on us for these specialized medicines." One month later, a federal grand jury indicted College Pharmacy on charges that it illegally imported and sold HGH from China. The 18-count indictment alleged that Bader and employee Kevin Henry—who obtained HGH from the Chinese company's sales rep, Bradley Blum—marketed the drug to at least four physicians.

Bader and Henry allegedly told physicians that because College was a compounding pharmacy, it wasn't subject to FDA regulations. Blum pled guilty to two counts and was sentenced to two years of probation and a $10,000 fine. After the pharmacy changed hands, the new owners agreed to forfeit $3.5 million as part of a government settlement. "Happily, crime still doesn't pay," said U.S. Attorney Troy A. Eid in a statement. Henry pled guilty to one count and was sentenced to one year of probation. Bader pled not guilty, but a jury found him guilty on most counts and he was facing sentencing in June 2010.

But there was an unresolved standoff between pharmacists and the FDA. It was a constant source of frustration for the FDA's Steve Silverman. And he saw only two possible resolutions. "Congress can amend our legislation to make it clear what it is they want the agency to do," he said. Or, alternatively, the FDA could petition the Supreme Court to revisit the issue. "As a general principal, the Supreme Court will often hear cases that involve conflicts between two federal circuits, so as to give clear guidance." But after weighing their options, Silverman and his colleagues opted against asking the Supreme Court for a resolution.

The FDA had to perform a delicate dance: It was trying to rein in compounders while at the same time maintaining a civilized dialogue with them. After the FDA responded to Wyeth's estriol petition in 2008—sending warning letters to seven pharmacies that were compounding the unapproved hormone—Silverman invited the IACP and several other pharmacy organizations to meet with him. During the gathering, which was held at the agency's Silver Spring, Maryland, headquarters, Silverman proposed that physicians wishing to prescribe estriol file investigational new drug (IND) applications. In so doing, those physicians would have to disclose safety information to patients, report any adverse events to the FDA, and agree to be monitored by an independent review board. Silverman told the pharmacists that the FDA would streamline the process for estriol—allowing single applications to cover multiple doctors and patients, for example.

Loyd Allen, who was there as an ambassador for the International Academy of Compounding Pharmacists, said that there were about a dozen FDA officials in the room talking up the IND plan. But he was not impressed. For physicians to apply for INDs, "they'd have to spend an excessive amount of time filling out government forms," said Allen, editor in chief of the *International Journal of Pharmaceutical Compounding*.

"They're not going to do that. We came to the conclusion that this plan was not workable."

Some who tried to go along with the FDA came to believe that the agency was merely setting traps. Rebecca Glaser, a doctor at the Millennium Wellness Center in Dayton, Ohio, wanted to treat women with testosterone and estriol in a study. So she filed an IND. The paperwork, which filled a one-inch binder, entailed hundreds of hours of work, she said. Then, in October 2008, an FDA agent showed up unannounced at Glaser's office and demanded to look at her patients' files. Later the agent visited the compounding pharmacies that Glaser used and warned them not to compound with estriol.

Glaser hired Houston lawyer Richard Jaffe, who had a reputation for getting pharmacists and doctors out of legal binds. He fired off a letter to the FDA, invoking the split in the circuit courts. "I believe the law in Ohio is that the Modernization Act is in force, and hence compounders can compound with estriol, which surely means that physicians can prescribe the product," he wrote. He informed the FDA that Glaser was withdrawing her IND and ordered the agency to cease its "abusive investigative tactic." Glaser and Jaffe didn't hear from the FDA again. Jaffe said the maze of legal decisions made it a challenge to counsel doctors, which he often did at anti-aging conferences. "They can't prescribe HGH for [anti-aging] under federal law, but can they prescribe estriol? I don't know," he said. "The FDA is trying to cut off the supply of estriol. They're trying to solve the problem that way. Can they intimidate people? For sure."

With every FDA action, the compounders only became more militant. In 2008, 340 pharmacists descended on Washington, D.C., for the IACP's 14th annual meeting, Compounders on Capitol Hill. They scheduled 300 get-togethers with congresspeople and persuaded two senators—John

Cornyn (R-TX) and Jim Bunning (R-KY)—to sponsor a Senate resolution calling on the FDA to reverse its estriol restrictions. "We applaud Sen. John Cornyn and Sen. Jim Bunning for their commitment to protecting hundreds of thousands of women," King said in a press release. "Women with menopause suffer enough. Fortunately, this resolution aims to provide them with some relief." IACP donated $3,000 to Cornyn during the 2008 election cycle, according to the Web site CampaignMoney.com (www.campaignmoney.com).

The blustery celebration of the senators' support was right in line with the compounding industry's MO: Pharmacists claimed to be looking out for the rights of patients, when they were seemingly protecting little more than their own bottom lines. In 2009, the National Community Pharmacists Association (NCPA) launched the Web site Fight4Rx (www.fight4rx.org). The site advertised itself as a "grassroots effort" to educate patients about the "value of their local community pharmacy," and the home page featured videos of pharmacists talking about their importance to their communities. Shortly after the site launched, NCPA's CEO Bruce Roberts claimed that it had already attracted 12,000 patients. But what those patients might not have realized was that NCPA was just another organization that relied on dues paid by compounding pharmacists.

It often looked as if compounders were trying to build support from local and federal lawmakers. Hotze funded a campaign against the Texas Medical Board, which he started after he published his book *Hormones, Health, and Happiness* in 2005. The board received anonymous complaints that Hotze was engaging in inappropriate advertising. Even though the case was dismissed, the investigation cost Hotze thousands in legal fees. "Hello? This is the United States of America. Hello? Of course I advertise," he said. "Drug companies are on TV every night. This stupid board doesn't have enough sense. Instead of going after bad doctors, they're worrying about whether or not I'm being successful." Hotze lobbied state legislators to pass a bill that would prohibit the medical board from using anonymous complaints and would require other measures to ensure doctors' "due process." (A bill containing many of Hotze's reform measures went nowhere in the Texas legislature.)

In 2006 and 2007, Hotze donated more than $2,500 to Texans for Senator John Cornyn, the cosponsor of IACP's estriol legislation. And on February 18, 2009, Hotze hosted a fund-raiser in his Houston home for Representative Joe Barton (R-TX), whom IACP labeled "a key ally." The event brought in $25,000.

The IACP had a knack for characterizing its fund-raising activities as education. In 2003, it started a nonprofit foundation and set out to raise $1.5 million to "fund research, educational alliances and public education." The foundation exceeded its goal, raising $2 million from donors such as PCCA, Medaus Pharmacy (a compounding pharmacy), and Gallipot. But the actual research was hard to find. IACP's Web site listed a handful of studies—but most were published in the compounding industry's own journals. A search on PubMed, the NIH's online database of medical articles, turned up zero IACP studies. Still, the money kept rolling in. IACP pulled in $1.7 million in membership fees and donations in 2006, much of which it funneled right back into lobbying. IACP paid out more than $71,000 in campaign contributions in the 2008 election cycle alone.

A few members of Congress resisted the compounders' efforts. On April 17, 2007, the Senate Committee on Aging held a hearing titled "Bio-identical Hormones: Sound Science or Bad Medicine?" Said Senator Larry Craig (R-ID) in his opening statement: "It concerns me that women who think they are choosing a natural alternative may not have all of the facts." Senator Gordon Smith (R-OR) held up a bottle of Natural Woman Progesterone Cream, which he said his staff had purchased on the Internet a few days earlier. "It comes with certain claims," Smith said. "Specifically that if applied topically, it will greatly decrease a woman's risk of breast cancer." He then asked panelist Jacques Rossouw, chairman of the Women's Health Initiative, if there were any studies to support such a claim. "No," Rossouw replied.

Smith bought the progesterone from one of 34 Web sites that had received warning letters from the FTC in 2005. The FTC had told site operators to stop claiming that progesterone could prevent and cure cancer, heart disease, or osteoporosis—or to provide evidence that such claims were true. Two years later, 32 of those sites were still up and running, and 19 were still making unsubstantiated claims. "You know, on the Western frontier, they had a lot of snake oil salesmen," Smith said. "Do we have that in the 21st century, if those claims are being made?"

Most of the panelists agreed with Craig and Smith, but there were two familiar faces who most definitely did not: Suzanne Somers's hormone expert T. S. Wiley and IACP spokesman Loyd Allen. Wiley, dressed in a purple suit and bifocals, sat forward in her chair and read a prepared statement. "Logically, if high circulating estrogen caused cancer, all young women would be dead; all pregnant women would be dead," she insisted, smirking and sighing to emphasize her points. "Now, the most recent move to keep us hormone-less is the debate over the value of compounded bio-identical hormones."

As for Allen, he may as well have been reading from the Old Testament of compounding. Pharmacists only prescribe hormones pursuant to individual prescriptions, he said, and the hormones "meet the needs of patients that are otherwise unmet by manufactured hormone products." Allen went on to promise that the compounding industry would consider establishing a database of safety information, where all pharmacists could go to print out detailed labels for each compounded product. No such database was ever implemented.

Senators Edward Kennedy (D-MA), Pat Roberts (R-KS), and Richard Burr (R-NC) drafted a bill called the Safe Drug Compounding Act of 2007. It proposed giving the FDA authority to inspect compounding pharmacies and to determine whether the products those pharmacists were selling were medically necessary or simply copies of commercially available drugs. The legislation also would have limited the intrastate sale of compounded drugs.

The compounding lobby kicked into high gear. Hotze responded by starting an organization called Project FANS (Freedom of Access to Natural Solutions). He started an online petition to Congress and announced a goal of collecting 100,000 signatures. "I don't like tyrants, injustice, regulatory agencies telling us what to do," he said at the time. "The FDA has been acting tyrannically and intrusively. They have no jurisdiction over us. They can't come in and try to put us out of business."

Nine pharmacy organizations, including the IACP and the National Community Pharmacists Association, sent a letter urging the senators not to introduce the bill. They scolded the senators for endangering patient care "by placing undue and counter-productive restrictions on licensed prescribers and pharmacists, while doing nothing to stop the rogue compounding practices that exist." The letter went on to tout the Pharmacy Compounding Accreditation Board as an example of the "great strides" the profession was taking to improve its practices. Compounders even recruited autism organizations to join the fight against the bill. Why? Because some parents of autistic children were fans of a fringe therapy known as "chelation," in which harsh chemicals were given by infusion to supposedly rid the body of mercury. Compounding pharmacies were major suppliers of chelation chemicals.

The Safe Compounding Bill never made it to the Senate floor. Two of the Senate's compounding critics left the Senate: Craig was arrested for lewd behavior in an airport bathroom and didn't run for reelection. Smith was voted out of office in 2008. The anti-aging industry and its merchants of hormones won time and again, especially in the court of public opinion. Even Hotze, after his legal misfires, was undaunted. He continued to recruit patients to his clinic and pharmacy, charging them $1,800 to $3,500 for a visit, plus $100 or so a month for hormones and supplements. "If I'm doing a good job, they will pay me," Hotze said. "And guess what? If I manage my money right, we'll make a profit. I feel like a million dollars."

The final score? Compounders: an estimated $2 billion in sales per year and growing. Regulators aiming to protect patients: zero.

Lawmakers, however, were determined to keep trying. In September 2008, the DEA issued a 198-count indictment against Midland Coalition member Applied Pharmacy Services. The indictment alleged that 12 executives, pharmacists, and dealers associated with the pharmacy illegally dispensed steroids, which were then distributed in virtually every state. Several doctors were also charged. As of early 2010, a jury handed guilty verdicts to five of the defendants. Four others were acquitted. Meanwhile, examples of careless compounding continued to come to light. In April 2009, Franck Pharmacy in Ocala, Florida, admitted to inadvertently making a superpotent veterinary mixture containing selenium, a supplement that can be poisonous in high doses. The medication was given to 21 elite polo horses. They all died.

Despite such tragedies, the compounding pharmacy industry powered ahead, largely unmonitored and strengthened by victories like that of the Loomises and Signature Compounding Pharmacy. The *Orlando Sentinel* reported that during a news conference at his Winter Park, Florida, pharmacy after the judge threw out the case, Stan Loomis declared, "The system worked." His troubles weren't over, however: in February 2010, the appellate division of the New York State Supreme Court ruled that the Albany County district attorney could present the charges to a new grand jury.

As the legal wrangling dragged on, those who most wanted the compounding industry to be shut down—the disgruntled consumer-protection advocates, the worried mothers—watched helplessly from the sidelines, crippled by their inability to build enough lobbying muscle to compete with outfits like IACP. "If you have money to promote bad science," said Sasich, "bad science prevails."

So does hypocrisy. Even as compounders continued to criticize big pharma for unethically marketing synthetic hormones, pharmacists began hiring high-priced sales representatives to market their own wares. On an e-mail subscriber list for compounders, a rollicking discussion broke out in 2009 on the value of hiring sales reps. One pharmacist reported that he had paid a rep $100,000 a year, plus benefits and expenses. Another pharmacist had two sales reps. Yet another posted this plea: "I know two people that are looking for a full-time marketing position for a compounding pharmacy. Please contact me off-line for contact information. (One person owned their own chemical company in another country before coming to the U.S.)" To the public, compounders continued to be their hometown heroes, offering specialized prescriptions to patients desperate for natural alternatives. But this online exchange told a different story: They could act just like pharmaceutical companies, but without any of the oversight needed to protect patients.

CHAPTER 8

Potions Galore

By the late 2000s, compounders had branched out big-time. Once they hooked patients on customized hormones, they found it easy to sell all sorts of pricey supplements and to claim that those supplements, too, were tailored to the unique needs of individual patients. Compounding Specialists of Wyoming, in Casper, for example, sold vitamin mixtures from a company called MyVitaminsRX. Claimed the pharmacy's Web site: "Based on the VitaminProfile, a unique metabolic test that opens a scientific window into your personal biochemistry, your customized MyVitaminsRX supplements are synergistically formulated for you and you alone from the most bioavailable forms of up to 50 critical nutrients." The cost? A mere $99.95 for a urine-testing kit, which promised to reveal exactly which vitamins a person should be taking, and in what ratios. Then patients paid a $69.95 monthly charge for an automatic shipment of vitamins supposedly formulated to match the test results.

There was no scientific reason to believe that a single urine sample could reveal an ideal vitamin formula for anyone. And there were no federal agencies monitoring companies like MyVitaminsRX to keep them honest. That's because the Dietary Supplement Health and Education Act (DSHEA) of 1994 shielded Signature, MyVitaminsRX, and other companies selling nutraceutical products. DSHEA left it completely up to manufacturers to determine whether the dietary supplements they made were safe and whether the marketing claims they spouted were backed up by adequate evidence. They were not required to provide the FDA or consumers with data about their products' safety or efficacy. And they didn't have to prove they were adhering to any federal standards of manufacturing.

As much as lax federal oversight allowed the anti-aging industry to get rich selling hormones and steroids, DSHEA provided an extra stimulus for extreme profiteering. DSHEA applied not just to vitamins but also to minerals, herbs, botanicals, amino acids, and even "glandulars"—ground-up glands from pigs or cows, which anti-aging doctors promoted as alternative sources of natural hormones. Physicians and pharmacies teamed up with nutraceutical manufacturers to market the potpourris, often persuading customers to hand over their credit card information so they could be charged automatically for monthly shipments.

The advertising claims were unrestrained. The label for AdvaClear, one of the 400 products sold by a BodyLogic nutritional supplier, Metagenics, claimed that it could provide "bifunctional support," which "enhances the activities of several hepatic detoxification enzymes while promoting balanced activity of the Phase I and Phase II detoxification pathways." The pill was basically a multivitamin, with extracts from green tea, artichokes, watercress, and pomegranate. Another Metagenics supplement, Cardiogenics, promised to deliver "minerals designed to be highly absorbable that play important roles in healthy heart muscle function through their involvement in nerve conduction and contraction and relaxation of the heart muscle." Among its ingredients: ground-up cow hearts.

Vitamins and minerals, and even beef by-products, are relatively safe. But they could cause extreme pain to people's pocketbooks. There was simply no reason to believe that designer supplements were worth paying ten times more for than one would pay for Centrum Silver, for example, which sold for as little as $3 a month. Yet many patients were fooled by boosterish language, such as that once displayed prominently on Signature's Web site: "In the timeless search for a true Fountain of Youth," it said, "customized nutritional supplementation has arrived and Signature Compounding Pharmacy is leading the way!"

It wasn't until the anti-aging industry threw dangerous chemicals into the mix that public health officials grew alarmed. As their stature in anti-aging circles grew, compounders began promoting chelation therapy, not just to cure autism but to prolong life. They combined the chelating agent ethylene-diamine-tetra-acetic acid (EDTA), a synthesized amino acid typically used to treat lead poisoning, with high-dose vitamins and minerals and distributed the preparations to anti-aging doctors to be used in intravenous treatments. Patients were told chelation would clear their bodies of dangerous chemicals, which in turn would protect their heart and other vital organs.

Such claims were based on scientifically flimsy reports that were out-of-date by about a half century. The FDA first approved

EDTA in 1953 to cure heavy metal poisoning, but some physicians noted that patients who had coronary artery disease felt better after the treatments. Virtually all the scientific papers on the phenomenon were case studies, however, rather than placebo-controlled trials, so chelation never caught on in cardiology.

Then, in 1973, a chelationist named Garry Gordon cofounded the American College for Advancement in Medicine (ACAM). He wrote a 12-page "position paper" on chelation therapy, heralding "widespread agreement that EDTA removes metallic catalysts which cause excessive oxygen free radical proliferation." Eliminating those catalysts, he claimed, "allowed the body's natural healing mechanisms to halt and often reverse the disease process." Most of the rest of the rambling document pointed to court cases that established the freedom to prescribe drugs off-label—cases that Gordon believed gave doctors a constitutional right to chelate.

In 1998, the FTC took note of ACAM's puffy marketing claims and charged the organization with false advertising. The agency questioned statements that appeared in ACAM's ads. "Every single study of the use of chelation therapy for atherosclerosis which has ever been published, without exception, has described an improvement in blood flow and symptoms," read one ad. In a settlement, ACAM agreed to stop making claims about the attributes of chelation in treating any disease of the human circulatory system, "unless supported by competent and reliable scientific evidence," an FTC statement said.

Nevertheless, chelation won over fans in high places. In her third book on anti-aging medicine, *Breakthrough*, Suzanne Somers declared chelation to be the magical detoxifier, capable of erasing decades of damage from eating too many mercury-filled tuna sandwiches and breathing in lead from pipes in homes and offices. "EDTA is three times less toxic than aspirin and has been tested and used safely for the past thirty years on an estimated half million patients . . . including me," she wrote. The aspirin statistic had been circulating in chelation circles for years, but it wasn't quite accurate. EDTA was known to be dangerous, especially if it was infused too rapidly. The risk was that EDTA would remove calcium ion from the blood more quickly than the body could replenish it. Calcium ion is vital for controlling heartbeat and other critical workings in the human body.

In fact, the Centers for Disease Control and Prevention (CDC) collected accounts of people who died while undergoing chelation, some of which were described in a 2006 *Journal of the American Medical Association* report. A 53-year-old Oregon woman with no history of heart disease was treated with EDTA provided by a compounding pharmacy, the CDC said. It was her fourth chelation session, and about 15 minutes into the treatment, she lost consciousness. She never woke up.

Retired psychiatrist Stephen Barrett was so perturbed he started a Web site called Chelation Watch (www.Chelation watch.org) in 2004 and began posting documents designed to debunk ACAM's claims. The site was an offshoot of Barrett's Quackwatch site (www.Quackwatch.org)—a repository for exposés of fringe treatments that Barrett thought were useless, dangerous, or both. In a paper on Chelation Watch, called "Chelation Therapy: Unproven Claims and Unsound Theories," biochemist Saul Green reviewed the handful of double-blind placebo-controlled studies that had been done on the procedure and concluded that none produced any noticeable improvement in heart health. Said Barrett, "There's neither any evidence, nor any logical reason to believe chelation works."

The biggest blow to the chelationists' cause was delivered by Quackwatch contributor and Tufts professor Kimball Atwood. The physician began digging up details about ACAM after he learned in 2003 that the NIH was starting a five-year, $30 million trial of chelation as a treatment for coronary artery disease. Atwood discovered that ACAM was one of the principal engineers of the protocol that would be used in the trial.

In 2008, Atwood posted an incriminating 72-page article in the online publication *Medscape Journal of Medicine*. In the document, titled "Why the NIH Trial to Assess Chelation Therapy (TACT) Should Be Abandoned," he claimed that several of the chelationists recruited to be coinvestigators in the trial had been disciplined by their state medical boards. Three were convicted felons. What's more, Atwood claimed, the consent form that patients signed was misleading. It said the FDA approved EDTA to treat lead poisoning, but not heart disease. In fact, according to Atwood, the type of EDTA used in the trial, called "disodium EDTA," wasn't approved even for treating lead poisoning. And in 2008, the FDA issued a safety alert, citing reports of children and adults who had died after they were given the drug. The two companies selling it withdrew it from the market.

The form went on to state that chelation had been "practiced in the community for many years" and that patients in the trial would "receive a standard intravenous mixture established by the American College for Advancement in Medicine." So the trial protocol was written by the organization that had the most to gain from a positive outcome—a conflict of interest that patients might not fully grasp, Barrett feared. "If consent is to be truly informed, it has to be based on real information," he said.

At one point, the password-protected Web site for the trial inexplicably became open to the public, allowing Atwood to read reports that investigators were filing. He discovered that two of the patients in the trial had died, he said. "It's not utterly clear the deaths had to do with chelation," Atwood said, "but incompetent medical care by chelationists was involved in both of them."

In September 2008, the NIH stopped recruiting new patients into the trial, pending an investigation by an independent review board. The trial's lead investigator, Gervasio Lamas, told a reporter for WebMD (www.webmd.com)—an online medical information provider—that he and his coinvestigators had taken Atwood's article seriously, convening several conference calls to discuss the allegations. They concluded that there was no reason to make any changes to the trial, though they did edit the consent form to clarify disodium EDTA's regulatory status. In a statement, ACAM said it would continue to work with Lamas to "answer the unfounded allegations of impropriety." But as far as Atwood was concerned, the patients who had already started the trial were in danger because they were still being treated with chelation. "My beef is not with ACAM," he said. "What bothers me is that NIH would get into bed with them."

Repurposing chemicals and using them to revive outmoded therapies was the anti-aging industry's new calling. Doctors moved from chelation to a whole host of bizarre chemical procedures that they believed could reverse deterioration all over the body. Some doctors offered "proliferative injection therapy," or "prolotherapy," as a cure for painful joints. Prolotherapy was invented in 1939 by a physician who believed that injecting chemicals such as dextrose directly into painful tendons and ligaments would cause new cells to grow—in essence allowing the body to heal itself. There was no scientific proof the treatment worked. The substances in prolotherapy injections were not approved by the FDA to treat bad backs and tennis elbows. But anti-aging was all about warding off the aches and pains of getting old, so predictably the industry revived prolotherapy and put it on their menus, right next to HGH and bio-identical hormone replacement.

Deborah Jennings decided to try prolotherapy after reading about it in Suzanne Somers's book *Ageless*. Jennings, a nurse in Rochester, New York, was suffering from arthritis in both hips. She found a doctor in nearby Williamsville who offered both bio-identical hormone-replacement therapy (BHRT) and prolotherapy. He persuaded Jennings that he could stop her hip joints from deteriorating any further. "If you shore up the ligaments and tendons, the joint will become stable and the disease process will be halted," Jennings said, recalling the doctor's advice. "The body rallies an immune response and recognizes it has a bigger problem and starts laying down collagen, which strengthens the ligaments."

But after six treatments, at a cost of $500 apiece, Jennings felt no relief at all. The doctor told her that with each injection, he could sense that her ligaments were starting to respond, and he convinced her to try three more treatments, she recalled. "Hard to know if he was just milking me along toward the end," she said. "I was hoping to stall surgery, but I was unable to do that."

Medicare deemed prolotherapy to be scientifically unverified, unreasonable, and unnecessary, and it refused to cover the treatment. Because Medicare sets the tone for the rest of the insurance industry, many of the nation's largest health plans followed suit with similar antiprolotherapy policies. In 1998, Aetna issued a policy bulletin on the procedure, seconding Medicare's position on prolotherapy, "because there is inadequate evidence of its effectiveness." It laid out a bevy of studies suggesting that prolotherapy was no better than saline injections for treating low-back pain.

New York physician Irwin Abraham was prolotherapy's most militant defender. The bearded, redheaded doctor explained how he performed the treatment in his Madison Avenue office. "The basic solution is dextrose, diluted with some lidocaine and water," he said, describing the potion as it was originally designed in the 1940s. "One of the old traditional ones, which is from England, is what's called 2PG, which stands for glycerin, phenol and glucose. You dilute that with water and some fat. It has a stronger kick." Abraham was a member of the American Association of Orthopaedic Medicine—which, like ACAM, was an organization that had an academic-sounding name but was a home for practitioners of alternative treatments.

In December 1997, Abraham requested that Medicare reverse its coverage policy on behalf of one of his patients. He backed up his petition with a scant five articles, only two of which were clinical trials. The agency rebuffed him. In one of the studies Abraham cited, the doctors had prescribed prolotherapy along with exercises, massages, and other treatments. That made it "difficult, if not impossible, to isolate the component of the treatment which gave the participants the reported relief," according to a 1999 Medicare coverage bulletin.

Even some of Abraham's own peers doubted that the therapy worked. Ten years after Medicare's decision, Charles Rosen, a professor of orthopedic surgery at the University of California at Irvine, took a look at the literature and found only 20 comprehensive studies of prolotherapy. Rosen was a passionate supporter of "evidence-based medicine"—the notion that all treatments should be backed up by definitive proof of their value to patients. In 2008, he founded the Association for Medical Ethics and began posting reviews of procedures, rating each one with a star system to reflect how well the research predicted the therapy would work. His verdict on prolotherapy wasn't pretty: For five different types of pain, on a scale of one to five stars, prolotherapy scored between one (very poor predictive ability for success of treatment) and three (fair predictive ability). Rosen posted the report on the Association for Medical Ethics Web site (www.ethicaldoctor.org) in 2009.

Abraham chalked up the criticism to professional jealousy. And he blamed the insurance industry for being closed-minded when it came to alternative treatments. "Basically," he said with a long sigh, "if you don't want to believe that something works, then no one can ever prove that it works."

Just uptown from Abraham, in an upscale Park Avenue clinic, yet another doctor was recommending chemical injections—this time seeming to promise that they would help patients regain the beauty of their youth. Marion Shapiro practiced "mesotherapy," a newfangled procedure that she said would melt fat. It was like liposuction but better, she said, because it wasn't quite so radical or invasive. Mesotherapy was hundreds of tiny injections of compounded medications, given in rapid succession with a "mesotherapy gun."

Shapiro's story, like that of so many anti-aging doctors, began in mainstream medicine. She started her career as an emergency room doctor in New Jersey. After her third son was born in 1998, she took a less demanding job as the manager of an urgent-care center. But she was bored. So when a friend made a passing reference to a French treatment called mesotherapy, Shapiro looked it up on the Internet. She couldn't find a single doctor performing the procedure in the United States. For Shapiro, this was an opportunity: She could introduce a new aesthetic product in one of the richest and most beauty-obsessed cities in the world. Shapiro flew off to Paris for a week, sought out a teacher, and spent two weeks learning the technique.

Shapiro's first patient was herself. She mixed up an asthma drug with some lidocaine, threw in a dash of vitamin C and caffeine, and turned the gun on her inner thighs. "I weighed 110 pounds, I worked out my whole life, but I could never lose my inner thigh fat," she said. "And guess what? I did. That's when I went from skeptic to believer."

Shapiro returned to the United States, opened her New York practice, and started booking appearances on TV shows popular with women, such as *The View*. "This is great," shouted co-host Joy Behar, introducing mesotherapy as the third installment in a 2003 series dubbed "Medical Miracles." "It claims to literally melt your fat away—hallelujah!" Shapiro stood next to Barbara Walters, a pointer in her hand. She showed photos of a woman who, after ten weeks of mesotherapy, lost four inches from her waist, hips, and thighs. The cost: $3,000. Immediately after the show aired, Shapiro got 595 calls from patients all over the country. "My practice exploded," Shapiro said.

The average patient watching the slim and distinguished Shapiro on TV might not have understood that mesotherapy didn't actually destroy fat cells. "After you release the fat from the patient, if she doesn't watch her weight, of course the fat comes back," said Shapiro, who seemed to have had no qualms about charging people thousands of dollars for what was, at best, a temporary fix.

The American Society of Plastic Surgeons (ASPS) wasn't convinced that mesotherapy was either safe or effective. In a 2008 "guiding principles" document it posted on its Web site, www.plasticsurgery.org, the organization warned that there were only 14 published trials on mesotherapy, 3 of which were poorly designed. None provided enough information on formulations and dosages. Some patients reported bruising and allergic reactions to the medications. Ultimately, the organization opted not to recommend mesotherapy.

ASPS spokesman Joe Gryskiewicz recalled discussing mesotherapy at the organization's annual Hot Topics meeting. The plastic surgeons in the group viewed before-and-after shots of a man who had mesotherapy injections in rolls of fat on his back. The rolls seemed to disappear. "It was miraculous," Gryskiewicz recalled thinking as the slides flashed on the screen. But then he realized that the man's arms were down by his side in the before photo, and straight up in the air in the after photo. "Everyone's back rolls get better when they put their arms up," Gryskiewicz said. "It's trash thrown out as good science."

Shapiro told her patients that all the medications she used were FDA approved. But they were not approved as fat-melting mixtures, so citing the FDA was misleading, critics said. Shapiro countered the concerns. "The FDA generally does not approve medications in combinations. The FDA does not regulate vitamins or herbal extracts, and that is definitely a big part of mesotherapy medication. So it really is about off-label use."

Why not design a double-blind placebo-controlled trial to boost mesotherapy's credibility? Shapiro's answer echoed a common response in the anti-aging community: "To do a proper study, you have to do MRIs, and probably biopsies," she said. "And you have to fund this. To do a correct, double-blind mesotherapy study would be costly."

She didn't need to do one anyway. By 2009, Shapiro had treated 5,000 patients, at a cost of about $550 per treatment. Demand was so high that she opened a second office in New Jersey. And it wasn't long before Shapiro had competition: She estimated that there were at least ten mesotherapists in every major metropolitan area by the end of the decade. Many of them started offering the treatment after just a few hours of training from operations that popped up to capitalize on the growing demand for the quick-fix fat burner.

Over time, the anti-aging industry became a giant vault for newly discovered disorders and their cures. One example was "adrenal fatigue," advanced by Arizona naturopath James Wilson. He noticed that many visitors to his Tucson clinic complained about similar patterns of listlessness. "They have tiredness in the morning. They don't feel like they slept well, even though they slept eight hours," he explained over lunch in a southwestern café near his office. "It takes them a while to wake up. They often need colas and coffee, something to stimulate them and keep them going during the day. They have an afternoon low. Some feel better after their evening meal—most do—but some people are spent by 8 o'clock."

Adrenal fatigue was known to mainstream doctors by a different name: normal adulthood. But the more Wilson studied his patients, the more convinced he became that he had hit on something that the entire field of endocrinology had overlooked. He believed that the adrenals—walnut-sized glands that sit on top of each kidney—could literally break down. Then they would stop pumping out essential hormones such as cortisol, which helps people heal when they get injured and calm themselves down when life's tribulations become overwhelming. The mounting responsibilities of work and family caused some people to run low on cortisol, Wilson surmised. "The reason most people get adrenal fatigue is because of lifestyle—burning the candle at both ends," he said.

Wilson's treatment regimen was much the same as what anti-aging doctors were recommending for HGH and bio-identical hormones. He tested the saliva of his patients, looking for what he thought was a telltale sign of adrenal fatigue: cortisol levels that drop precipitously throughout the day. He believed that if he replaced cortisol, using the steroid hydrocortisone, the adrenal glands would be propped up. Once the adrenals were able to get some rest, they could kick back in and work normally again, he said.

Hydrocortisone was generally used to treat inflammatory diseases such as rheumatoid arthritis and serious glandular conditions such as Cushing's syndrome and Addison's disease. But Wilson believed people with not-so-well-defined illnesses could benefit from it, too. "I typically recommend people start with 5 milligrams in the morning. If they have difficulty getting out of bed, I tell them to keep it right by their bedside and take it with salted water," to relieve the salt cravings that adrenal fatigue commonly caused, he explained. "About noon they may need another 2.5 to 5 milligrams. And then at 4 they may need another 1.5 to 2 milligrams, and they might need 1 to 2.5 milligrams before they go to bed." His notion that supplementing with hydrocortisone would help the adrenal glands recover came from "a couple of papers that appeared in the '60s," he said.

Wilson began preaching about adrenal fatigue at gatherings for natural-medicine practitioners. In 1994, Klatz and Goldman invited him to speak at one of their first conferences in Las Vegas, and he returned year after year. Wilson wasn't sure how he ended up on A4M's radar, but he was more than willing to train new anti-aging recruits. In 2001, he published a book called *Adrenal Fatigue: The 21st Century Stress Syndrome.*

A4M's Pamela Smith recruited Wilson to be a faculty member in the anti-aging fellowship program. During lectures at A4M's conferences, Wilson urged fledgling anti-aging doctors to think about stress as a problem worth solving with medications. "I talked about how important stress is to our society—how expensive it is to businesses," he said. His book became required reading in anti-aging circles. By 2007, it was in its 11th printing, and Wilson was making enough of a living as a teacher and author to quit seeing patients.

But what Wilson was teaching ran counter to what centuries of research had proven to be true of stress and adrenal function. Everyone's cortisol levels look low in saliva samples at any given time, particularly in the afternoon. When cortisol levels are dangerously low, the pituitary gland produces more of a substance called adrenocorticotropic hormone (ACTH). The whole cascade can be measured with an intricate series of injections and blood tests, which endocrinologists considered to be essential for diagnosing an adrenal problem that truly needed to be treated. "You cannot have low adrenal function if your ACTH level is normal," said Leonard Wartofsky, a Georgetown professor and chairman of the department of medicine at Washington Hospital Center.

Wilson mentioned ACTH testing as an option in *Adrenal Fatigue* but brushed it off as generally unnecessary. He insisted the condition could be spotted from saliva tests and symptoms alone. His book even gave patients tools for diagnosing themselves. One was a long questionnaire, consisting of a series of statements, which readers were asked to rate on a scale of 0 ("never/rarely") to 3 ("intense/severe or frequent"). "My sex drive is noticeably less than it used to be," read one statement. "My thinking is confused when hurried or under pressure," read another.

Despite the questions swirling around the reliability of saliva testing and questionnaires as diagnostic tools, doctors continued to find that patients were suffering from adrenal fatigue. BodyLogic's chief medical officer, Alicia Stanton, recalled one 41-year-old man who came in complaining of no particular symptoms. He just wanted to make sure his health was optimal. "I looked at his labs. His adrenals were horrible," said Stanton, referring to his chart, which showed his cortisol levels dropping throughout the day. "I said, 'You don't have symptoms, but I look at this and I don't know how you're getting through your day.'" Stanton pushed a little harder, asking him to recall feelings or behaviors that might fit the adrenal-fatigue template. "He said, 'Well actually I'm kind of dragging; I hit the snooze a couple times.'" He became a new patient.

Hydrocortisone is not the type of drug that should be handed out like aspirin, not even in tiny doses. It raises the risk of diabetes, osteoporosis, hypertension, and infertility. Wilson admitted that it can be addictive because it produces an intoxicating high. "Once you get them to a certain treatment level they're feeling good," he said. "They don't like to give that up. Meanwhile their heart is being eaten away, their eyes are deteriorating, their liver's having problems. We don't want them to get into that kind of a cortisol-addicted state."

Wilson also recommended less drastic treatments for adrenal fatigue, too. He championed extracts from cow glands, for example, which were once used to treat adrenal disorders. In his book, Wilson blamed the drug industry for causing bovine extracts to fall out of favor because it was more profitable for them to sell hydrocortisone. It was an argument similar to what proponents of bio-identical hormones were saying. But it wasn't widely supported by science. Doctors favored synthetic cortisol because it was engineered to mimic what the body made naturally—making it far more effective and potent than cow extracts.

Thyroid hormone, a treatment for disorders of the thyroid gland, provided another example of seemingly bizarre anti-aging logic. When anti-aging doctors diagnosed low thyroid, they often prescribed a product made of dried, ground-up pig glands to treat it. It was called Armour, and it was akin to the drugs that were used to treat thyroid problems in the first half of the 20th century. One day in 2009, a patient called Stanton to ask a logical question: Why is pig thyroid good but horse estrogen bad? Because, Stanton answered, Armour is closer to what our bodies make naturally.

The anti-aging industry's infatuation with Armour may not have been well grounded in science, Wartofsky said. In the

1950s, the drug companies learned how to make chemical copies of the body's own natural thyroid. Most doctors stopped prescribing the pig version, for good reason. Normally our bodies take a form of thyroid called T4 and convert it to T3. Synthetic thyroid, known as thyroxine, is a chemical copy of T4, which the body converts to T3 naturally. Armour, on the other hand, contains both forms of thyroid—and that can cause a dangerous overdose of T3. "When you take Armour Thyroid, your T3 level goes up acutely," Wartofsky said. "In older patients, this may cause atrial fibrillation, arrhythmias. Even in younger patients it may cause headaches, because it produces too rapid a rise in thyroid hormone levels."

Many anti-aging doctors redefined the word "low" in diagnosing low thyroid. Most people who have mild symptoms of low thyroid—fatigue, dry skin, cold hands and feet, forgetfulness—actually have completely healthy thyroids. Nonetheless in addition to performing the test for thyroid-stimulating hormone, which is used to detect low thyroid, some anti-aging doctors measured another molecule called "reverse T3." Invariably a patient with normal levels of thyroid-stimulating hormone would turn out to have abnormal amounts of reverse T3—which gave doctors a reason to treat patients that many physicians would regard as healthy. According to Wartofsky, the role of reverse T3 in the human body is unclear. "As far as we know, it has no metabolic function," said Wartofsky. "It's simply created, broken down and destroyed."

Many anti-aging doctors also started promoting DHEA as a solution for adrenal fatigue and as a ward against cardiovascular disease and cancer. DHEA was a banned steroid until 1994's dietary supplement legislation reclassified it as a nutritional product. DHEA pills began showing up in health food stores everywhere, at prices as high as $30 a bottle.

But most of the supposedly wonderful benefits of the hormone were claims that came out of uncontrolled trials or case reports. And there was evidence that DHEA could increase the risk of cholesterol problems and breast and ovarian cancer. In 1999, two endocrinologists from the University of British Columbia reviewed every study on DHEA they could find and published their impressions in a paper called "DHEA: Panacea or Snake Oil?" in the journal *Canadian Family Physician*. It's clear which of the two they deemed DHEA to be. "Current enthusiasm for using DHEA as a panacea for aging, heart disease, and cancer is not supported by scientific evidence in the literature," they wrote. "Given the potentially serious adverse effects, using DHEA in the clinical setting should be restricted to well-designed clinical trials only."

Perhaps the oddest therapy that the anti-aging industry promoted was progesterone for men. Anti-aging doctors believed that when people were stressed-out, their bodies would make so much cortisol that they wouldn't be able to make all the other hormones. Hence the need for hydrocortisone, as well as for bio-identical hormone replacement, they told their patients. But why did men need progesterone, a female sex hormone? Doctors and pharmacists claimed that it would help revive the adrenals, which would benefit men's hearts and prostates.

It is true that the male body makes progesterone, which then converts to cortisol, but most doctors say the hormone doesn't really do much beyond that. Even some anti-aging doctors were appalled when they started seeing their industry promote progesterone for men. Neal Rouzier, who practiced anti-aging medicine in Palm Springs, California, cringed when a presenter at the 2009 Age Management Medicine Group conference in Boca Raton recommended prescribing progesterone to protect against prostate cancer. "There is no evidence progesterone protects the prostate, and there are two studies that say it's harmful," said Rouzier during a break from the presentations.

In his own lecture at the conference, Rouzier begged his peers to follow the evidence. "Can anyone tell me why estriol is safe?" he said, citing the female hormone that had grown so popular because of anti-aging promotions. "I think it's one of the unsafest hormones. Prescribe estradiol. It will convert to estriol."

Rouzier believed his propensity to speak out against the industry's most lucrative products got him banished from A4M conferences. "It's very ridiculous," Rouzier said. "It's about politics and economics." Still, Rouzier refused to be silenced, calling himself "the messenger boy" for the scientific literature. "My criticism of these groups is that so much of what they teach and do is not evidence-based," he said, glancing over his shoulder and speaking in a quiet hush so as not to offend the conference's organizers. "Our critics say we're quacks. I sort of agree. But I'm trying to be pure science."

Science has, on occasion, produced evidence that some supplements—especially vitamins—can ease the aging process. In 2009, a group of Harvard scientists published results from an eight-year study showing that vitamin B and folic acid can prevent the eye disease known as age-related macular degeneration in some patients. It was just the type of study that was sorely lacking in the anti-aging industry: It was lengthy, double-blind, and placebo-controlled. And it was huge, with more than 5,000 patients enrolled.

Anti-aging doctors commonly cried poor, claiming that they didn't have the funding necessary to run such trials. But it's more likely that the industry was hiding from the truth. If any rigorous scientific study showed that anti-aging therapies were ineffective or unsafe—and that they didn't truly extend life—the industry would be dead.

CHAPTER 9

Anti-Aging Goes Mainstream

On January 11, 2008, TV chef and talk show maven Rachael Ray sipped from a cup of MonaVie, a dark purple drink made of 19 fruits, including the Brazilian berry açaí. MonaVie was the featured product that day in "The Dish with Lara Spencer," a weekly segment on *Rachael Ray* featuring Spencer, cohost of the Hollywood tabloid show *The Insider*. "MonaVie is probably the healthiest drink you can get," raved Spencer. "This is Oprah Winfrey's super genius smart food of all smart foods," she continued. Spencer revealed that MonaVie cost $45 a bottle, eliciting a stunned "Whoa!" from Ray. But it was worth it, Spencer insisted. "It apparently increases your memory; it helps fight off heart disease," she said. "All the people in the know are drinking it."

The MonaVie company was founded in 2005 by Dallin Larsen, a Utah-based entrepreneur. The company was like the Amway of anti-aging, employing independent salespeople to hawk the potion to friends, family, and doctors. They marketed

MonaVie as a powerful antioxidant that could curb cancer and high cholesterol, control weight, and soothe aches and pains. By 2009, Larsen claimed he had sold $1 billion worth of the juice and had signed on his millionth sales rep. And MonaVie had Hollywood street cred: It garnered raves not just from Ray but from the likes of 85-year-old Viacom CEO Sumner Redstone, who predicted it would help him live another 50 years. At a 2008 MonaVie sales meeting in Anaheim, California, the bald, suited Larsen paced the stage and bellowed, "I do believe we've got the product, the timing, the management, the compensation plan and cause to make this the largest direct-selling company in the history of the planet earth."

It had been about a dozen years since Klatz and Goldman conceived of A4M at the El Dorado longevity clinic in Cancun, and the unquenchable desire to fight off aging had infiltrated every aspect of American life. Anti-aging entrepreneurs were everywhere, latching on to just about anything—fruits, vitamins, herbs, vegetables—and claiming they paved the path to the fountain of youth. The line between science and anti-aging hucksterism had completely blurred. Talk show hosts were doctors. Businesspeople were healers. And patients were so desperate to believe they could turn back the clock that they rarely questioned whether the remedies being recommended to them were backed up by rigorous science—or whether it was all just one big illusion.

Nowhere was the full splendor of the anti-aging medicine chest more evident than at A4M's massive conferences. At the 2008 Las Vegas shindig, entrepreneurs selling all manner of packaged youth tossed out samples and sales pitches from booths lined up along nine sprawling aisles. Supplement makers such as DaVinci Laboratories of Essex Junction, Vermont, offered to custom manufacture vitamins and then private-label them for anti-aging doctors. BioPharma Scientific of San Diego was showing off NanoGreens[10], a $49.95 canister filled with a drink mix that purportedly delivered the nutritional punch of ten fruits and vegetables. Med Mar, Inc., offered "the miracle of medical marijuana"—nonprescription gelcaps that could supposedly lower cholesterol, relieve arthritis pain, and stabilize blood sugar. "Now legal in 50 states," bragged the company's brochure. (Its product was really just an extract of the cannabis seed used to grow marijuana.) MonaVie was there, too, in a large booth where company representatives persuaded doctors to sell the juice out of their offices, promising they could earn 100 percent profit margins on each sale.

Açaí was the premier example of an anti-aging elixir gone completely out of control. The açaí berry, which is about the size of a grape, is native to the Brazilian Amazon, where for centuries it has been consumed as juice, a salad ingredient, and even made into a liqueur. It wasn't discovered by Americans until the end of the 20th century, when alternative-health advocates embraced so-called functional foods—edible delicacies thought to provide much more than good taste and basic nutrition. Açaí started showing up in juices such as MonaVie and as extracts in supplements sold in health food stores. Millions of Internet ads popped up on consumer sites and in Google searches for anything "aging."

As the berry grew more and more popular, the claims grew wilder. Some açaí sellers said it could enhance eyesight and promote a healthier metabolism; others referred to it as nature's Viagra. In 2007, the FDA sent a letter to one Texas distributor, admonishing him for marketing MonaVie as if it were a drug. The letter pointed to language on his Web site that suggested açaí could relieve muscle pain and that claimed it "also contains many valuable Phytosterols. Sterols are compounds of plant cell membranes providing numerous benefits to the Human body, namely the reduction of blood plasma cholesterol." The FDA pointed out that MonaVie's products were not recognized as safe or effective for such conditions and therefore could not be legally marketed that way without approval.

Two years later, other açaí sellers were still making outrageous claims, prompting the Washington, D.C.–based Center for Science in the Public Interest to issue a public warning. David Schardt, a nutritionist at the center, said there was no evidence the extract could cleanse colons, enhance sexual desire, or perform other miracles. He found only a handful of studies of the fruit, which did show that eating it causes antioxidant levels in the blood to rise. "But that's true for every fruit," he said. "These companies are exaggerating the benefits." Schardt discovered more than 75 açaí-related blogs, with names like "Olivia's Weight Loss Blog" and "Becky's Weight Loss Blog," all of which claimed to be first-person accounts of the fruit's remarkable slimming powers. But Olivia, Becky, and all the other women were actually the same German model, and the blogs were nothing more than ad copy. "Fake blogs," marveled Schardt. "Shameless."

The Better Business Bureau of Utah gave MonaVie a C rating after it received more than 45 complaints about the company's billing, sales, and service practices. But its distributors continued to stretch the truth in their ads: When one claimed that Brad Pitt was a fan of the product, the actor's lawyer called the company with a warning to stop using Pitt's name. He didn't drink MonaVie.

Açaí juice wasn't the only liquid that touched off an anti-aging free-for-all. In 2003, Harvard scientist David Sinclair announced that resveratrol, a substance found in red wine, seemed to promote longevity. Wine connoisseurs buzzed that the discovery might explain the "French paradox," the puzzling fact that people in France live long, healthy lives, even as they wolf down foie gras and other fatty delicacies. At a scientific meeting in the Swiss Alps in the summer of 2003, the youthful-looking Australian scientist could barely contain his excitement, telling the *New York Times*, "I've been waiting for this all my life." Sinclair hadn't done enough research to be able to say confidently that resveratrol had any therapeutic value for people. Nonetheless, he told the *Times*, "One glass of red wine a day is a good recommendation. That's what I do now."

Unlike açaí, resveratrol actually had a scientific pedigree. Sinclair's finding stemmed from research he had started in 1991 while working with aging expert Leonard Guarente of the Massachusetts Institute of Technology. Guarente discovered that starving yeast lived longer than well-fed yeast and that a gene called *sir2* modulated the longevity response. Tests in mice confirmed the finding with stunning results: Cutting 30 percent of calories seemed to extend life by as much as 30 percent.

But chopping out a third of the human diet would be unbearable—indeed, inhumane—so scientists such as Sinclair started searching for drugs that might turn on the longevity gene. Sinclair tested hundreds of chemicals, hoping to find just one that would modulate sirtuin, an enzyme produced by the gene. Resveratrol was a perfect match.

In 2004, Sinclair cofounded (with Christoph Westphal) the biotech company Sirtris Pharmaceuticals, and it became an instant Wall Street darling. Sirtris raised $60 million in a flashy 2007 stock market debut. Less than a year later, GlaxoSmithKline bought the startup for $720 million—an enormous premium considering that Sirtris was years away from getting any product on the market. By that time, Sirtris had already moved on from resveratrol, developing synthetic drugs that would activate the same life-extending gene but in a much more powerful way.

Because the FDA didn't classify aging as a disease, Glaxo wasn't studying the drugs for that purpose. Instead, it was testing them to treat diseases common in older people, such as cancer and diabetes. Anti-aging folks would fall back on an old argument and say the companies weren't developing resveratrol because natural substances can't be patented. The reality was that resveratrol wasn't very potent; it never would have cut it as a serious therapy.

These nuances were completely lost on the mainstream media, however. Barbara Walters featured Sinclair in a 2008 ABC News TV special called *Live to Be 150 . . . Can You Do It?* As Walters and Sinclair toasted each other with red wine, Walters asked how many glasses she would have to drink to get the anti-aging benefits. "A thousand bottles a day," he answered, eliciting a humorous smirk from Walters. Sinclair also appeared with Sirtris cofounder Westphal on *60 Minutes.* Westphal shook out some unidentifiable caplets into his hand as correspondent Morley Safer raved, "We all might soon be taking a drug that just might beat the clock—a simple pill that could delay the inevitable." Sinclair said, "The important news here is not that we found something in red wine. The important thing is we passed a milestone where we can now make drugs based on this knowledge and potentially slow down aging itself."

The irresistible notion of encapsulating 1,000 bottles of red wine or a miraculous berry extract gave rise to a whole new class of anti-aging entrepreneurs. Companies such as FWM Laboratories of Hollywood, Florida, began selling açaí and resveratrol pills, which they marketed on the Web through ads served up by Google, Yahoo, and other search engines.

These companies painted the media attention as big-time endorsements for their products. Oprah Winfrey and her resident doctor, Mehmet Oz, talked up açaí and resveratrol on Winfrey's shows but didn't endorse any specific products. Still, supplement makers attached those clips to their ads, right next to claims such as this one for FWM's Resveratrol Ultra: "Resveratrol Ultra is one of the most popular products. It has been featured over and over again on *60 Minutes*, the Dr. Oz show, CNN, NBC and *The New York Times*." (It had not.) Ads disseminated through search engines contained links with titles such as "Dr-sinclair-resveratrol.com." Consumers who clicked on the ads were brought to pages that offered free trials and that replayed Sinclair's appearances on *60 Minutes* and ABC. "If you have been following *60 Minutes*, you would have seen my segment on resveratrol, and everything it can do for you," read the ad's text beside a photo of Sinclair. "As mentioned, I take resveratrol myself, and love it."

The sites offered free trials to everyone who typed in a credit card number. Those who tried to click off the Sinclair ads were stopped by a large boxed message, which read, "Wait! Dr. Sinclair wants to make sure you take advantage of this limited time opportunity!" Another link to a similar ad was labeled "Sirtris Official Site," even though the product featured in the ad had never been endorsed by Sinclair, Sirtris, or Glaxo.

The supplement sellers promised free trials of açaí and resveratrol. But what they really did was surreptitiously sign customers up to receive automatic shipments costing upward of $80 a month. Buried in the fine print were notices that customers had 15 days to cancel and that the trial period would start as soon as they typed in their credit card numbers—not when they received the products. Many customers complained that they didn't even get their shipments until well after their 15-day free-trial period had passed. Buyers who tried to get out of the subscriptions found that they couldn't reach customer-service departments by phone or e-mail. Some had to cancel their credit cards just to break free from the schemes. The consumer site Complaints Board (www.complaintsboard.com) collected more than 17,000 posts from furious buyers of açaí and resveratrol.

Within months of the supplements' introduction, scam artists had developed all sorts of wily ways to sell them. One ad pitching several brands of resveratrol, including FWM's, displayed a full-page testimonial from Katie Wilson, a health reporter for a local news station in California. Wilson wrote that after taking resveratrol for 30 days, she had softer skin, thicker hair, and more energy. But Katie Wilson didn't exist. She was fictional, and she turned up again in a nearly identical testimonial, this time as a reporter for "News Channel 9," also fake. Some of the most audacious supplement sellers went so far as to lure in customers by claiming they were actually shielding them from scams. One Resveratrol Ultra ad, for example, read, "Warning! Want to Use Resveratrol, Read This Warning." Oddly enough, the so-called warning popped up frequently on Complaints Board, while consumers were searching for forums on FWM's atrocious marketing practices.

Even when serious scientists tried to dampen the hype, they inadvertently fed into it, almost as if they wanted to believe it themselves. Long after Sinclair conceded that resveratrol wasn't very effective, he continued to show videos of his resveratrol-fed mice running endlessly on a treadmill. "It's not that they can run farther," he told a group of journalists at the

International Longevity Center in New York in 2009. "It's that they look metabolically as if they've been exercising." The longest-lived mouse in his experiments, he said, made it to age three—a year older than rodents are expected to live.

Sinclair once served on the scientific advisory board of Shaklee Corporation, a Pleasanton, California, company that sold Vivix Cellular Anti-Aging Tonic, which contained resveratrol. For a short time, his photo appeared on some Vivix promotional material. But he became disturbed when other companies started latching on to him, too, so he quit the Shaklee post. "I don't want to overpromise," Sinclair conceded. "I don't want to be the guy doing the equivalent of cold fusion." Sinclair estimated that humans would have to take up to five grams of resveratrol a day to get the same benefits seen in the mice. That's a lot of pills, especially when you consider that one dose of Resveratrol Ultra, for example, was just 62.5 milligrams.

Nevertheless, the supposed celebrity endorsements fooled tens of thousands of youth-seeking consumers. Himani Vejandla, a Ph.D. student in physiology at West Virginia University, ordered what she thought was a free trial of Resveratrol Ultra in 2009. She was reading an article on the medical-information site WebMD when the ad popped up, and she was impressed that experts such as Sinclair and Oz supposedly endorsed the product. But she got suspicious when the shipment arrived with no information about how to return the pills. Then FWM double-charged her $87.13. She had to file a claim with her bank to try to recover the second payment after FWM's customer-service people told her they had no record of the charge. "They're literally ripping people off," Vejandla said.

Colleen Florio, a psychologist in Glens Falls, New York, read the terms and conditions carefully before she ordered FWM's supplements, and she knew full well she would have to return them in 15 days. But she didn't receive her shipment until the 15th day. "They made it impossible to send it back," Florio said. "I was flabbergasted. I must have called ten times." Florio was particularly puzzled because she saw the ad when she was reading an article on Oprah's Web site, so she thought the talk show host had, in fact, endorsed the supplements. "Oprah wouldn't advertise a product if it wasn't good," she said.

Because the Internet is largely unregulated, supplement makers found it remarkably simple to propagate scams. Most didn't write or place their own ads on the Web but instead worked through networks of advertising "affiliates," which they paid to spread the word about their products through Google, Yahoo, and other sites. FWM CEO Brian Weiss said that his affiliates wrote the ads for his products and that when he got wind of inappropriate celebrity endorsements, he instructed them to take the ads down immediately. Lawyers for the celebrities did plenty of griping, but the effort to control the fictional celebrity endorsements was like a big game of Whac-A-Mole: As soon as one fishy ad came down, another went up, with a different URL.

A 2009 change in Google's policies made it even easier for FWM and its rivals to further pursue their marketing strategies. The search company relaxed its policies governing how advertisers could use trademarks in its popular AdWords program. Through AdWords, companies bid on the placement of their promotions in searches and sponsored links and paid only when Web surfers clicked on their ads. The program accounted for most of Google's $22 billion in annual revenues. Google's new policy was sure to boost AdWords' popularity because it allowed companies to cite registered trademarks in ads, even if they didn't own those trademarks. The point was to enable legitimate commerce: An online shoe store, for example, could drive more traffic to its site by using trademarked names like Nike and Adidas in its AdWords copy.

But Google was supposed to prohibit advertisers from making false claims and from pushing credit card fraud schemes. And it used both automated and manual processes to catch violators before their ads were posted. Oprah and Rachael Ray are trademarked names, making them particularly vulnerable to false advertising. When a Google spokeswoman was asked why so many faux celebrity endorsements were making it through the AdWords filters, she could only answer helplessly, "We're doing our best."

The FTC was slow to catch on to anti-aging scams, even though it was clearly on the prowl for illegal Internet cons. In early 2009, the FTC asked Google and Facebook to pull down ads claiming to offer consumers money from President Barack Obama's stimulus plan. In July of that year, the agency brought eight cases against companies using the Web to market get-rich schemes and money-saving opportunities that turned out to be nothing more than excuses for them to collect credit card numbers. The agency would neither confirm nor deny that it was investigating supplement makers, but FTC attorney Karen S. Hobbs said that it didn't look kindly on CEOs who said, as Weiss did, that it was affiliate ad networks that were responsible for false claims. "Our position is, companies cannot hide behind affiliate marketing. We pursue companies directly," she said.

Florida's Better Business Bureau (BBB), which was flooded with complaints, slapped FWM with an F rating. Weiss said that the customer-service gripes about FWM were "older complaints" and that the company had put in place 24-7 phone and Web support to alleviate the problems. He said he answered every BBB complaint. CBS News, which also investigated FWM, tracked down Weiss at his warehouse, where dozens of workers were furiously packing up pills as printers churned out reams of mailing labels. Weiss told the reporter that his company contacted unhappy customers and that the volume of complaints was actually small compared to the many thousands of customers the company had attracted. But Michael Galvin, a spokesman for the BBB in Miami, said that none of that mattered. "We have serious concerns about his sales techniques. He'll still have an F."

State attorney generals soon stepped in. The Florida attorney general's Economic Crimes Division in West Palm Beach launched an investigation of FWM in 2009. And Connecticut attorney general Richard Blumenthal announced that he was working with officials in other states to investigate the business practices of companies selling açaí. "There are no magical berries from the Brazilian rainforest," Blumenthal said in a statement, "only painfully real credit card charges."

Even Winfrey—who not only championed anti-aging hormones, but also featured Oz as a frequent expert on staying young—had enough. She warned fans with two postings on her Web site: "Consumers should be aware that neither Oprah Winfrey nor Dr. Oz are associated with nor do they endorse any açaí berry product, company or online solicitation of such products, including MonaVie juice products," read one. "Neither Oprah Winfrey nor Dr. Oz are associated with nor do they endorse any specific resveratrol product, company or online solicitation of such products," said another.

In August 2009, Winfrey's and Oz's production companies filed suit against more than 50 supplement sellers and their affiliate advertisers, including FWM. Among the allegations: trademark and copyright infringement, false endorsement, and "cybersquatting," the use of domain names that were "confusingly similar" to those used by Winfrey and Oz. The complaint included screen shots of ads, some of which were identical to the Sinclair ads but containing Oz's photo instead. "I take resveratrol myself, and love it," said one Oz ad. The words "as seen on Oprah" were included on a banner at the bottom. Marc Rachman, an attorney with Davis & Gilbert in New York, which handled the suit, said, "They are not authorized to use clips from the show. They are not authorized to use the names and likenesses. The ads are purporting to talk in Dr. Oz's voice. Customers thought he was endorsing these supplements. This is deceptive and it is a false endorsement." Rachman's grandest wish for the suit, he said, was not so much to win damages for Winfrey and Oz. "We want consumers to get their money back."

Noel Patton was a retired appliance-manufacturing executive who joined A4M shortly after its inception. He had just turned 50, he said, and "I started to feel the effects of aging. I didn't like it so well." At a charitable dinner in Texas in 1999, Patton heard a professor lecture on telomerase, an enzyme that seemed to make cells immortal. Scientists believed telomerase lengthened telomeres, DNA sequences that sat on the ends of chromosomes and protected them from destruction. The longer the telomeres, scientists thought, the lower the risk for developing age-related diseases. Patton pulled the professor aside and told him, "I'm really interested. How do I get some of these immortal cells?" The professor laughed and told Patton they had all been licensed to a company called Geron.

The next day, Patton called the CEO of Geron, a publicly held San Francisco biotech company that was renowned for its work with stem cells. Geron had discovered a substance from the Chinese herb astragalus that seemed to activate telomerase, but its scientists had shelved it. Instead, they were pursuing the idea that inhibiting telomerase (rather than stimulating it) might actually help treat diseases such as cancer. Nevertheless, Patton asked if he could license the astragalus-derived substance and turn it into an herbal supplement—a request that made Geron executives balk at first. "I had no science background, no medical background, and these are Ph.D.'s and M.D.'s," Patton said. "I had no company, no infrastructure, so they wondered how could I do something like this? I convinced them that maybe I would be an OK candidate." Patton started up a company in Manhattan and called it TA Sciences, for "telomerase activation."

In 2002, Geron licensed the telomerase activator to Patton's company. TA Sciences spent five years developing an astragalus extract from three tons of the plant, harvested in Mongolia. Patton started taking it himself, and in 2007 he began to sell it as a nutraceutical called TA-65. But he didn't sell it in individual bottles or even on the Internet by subscription. Instead, he required that everyone who wanted to try it enroll in his "Patton Protocol," at a cost of $25,000 for the first year. Customers who signed on agreed to take TA-65 along with 55 vitamins and minerals and to have more than 90 blood tests every six months. In two years, 100 customers signed up to try the protocol.

Despite the appearance of scientific rigor, there was no way to truly prove that TA-65 lengthened telomeres. And as Patton sat in his well-appointed upper-East-Side office two years after launching the protocol, he tried to explain the $25,000-per-year price tag. Telomere length changes so slowly, he said, that "this test is not that accurate when you compare six-month intervals." Nevertheless, he claimed, his customers were seeing an improvement in "the immune system and a number of other things." He pointed to a scientific experiment in Spain in which mice given a telomerase activator (not TA-65) lived 24 percent longer than normal mice. "I don't want to exaggerate or whatever, but I feel younger now and more energetic and quicker than I did when I started all this," Patton said. "There's a plethora of anti-aging products out there, and they're all BS and snake oil. If you feel better and look better, that's important."

The next day, Patton flew off to Florida to display TA-65 at A4M's Miami conference and then at Age Management Medicine Group's competing Boca Raton event. He handed out brochures with pictures of TA Sciences' clients, including a 70-year-old dad who was shown kissing his newborn child's forehead. "Independent tests have verified that TA-65 can significantly improve several key parameters of aging, including immune structure, bone density and mental function," the brochure promised. Buried in the fine print was this disclaimer: "These statements have not been evaluated by the Food and Drug Administration. This product is not intended to diagnose, treat, cure or prevent any disease."

So why did people continue to believe? Why were they so eager to give their credit card numbers to companies like FWM or to fork over thousands of dollars for questionable prescriptions from an expanding collection of doctors? Because in the quest for eternal youth, they refused to consider that the magic bullets—the supplements, syringes, tinctures, and tonics— might be useless, or worse, dangerous. So eager were they to take an express train back to their prime that they believed a

15-day free trial would give them enough time to determine if the latest anti-aging cure-all was truly making them younger.

Most of all, they were unable to accept that the only proven route to longevity required giving up the foods they loved and sweating through frequent workouts. Exercise is probably the only anti-aging regimen that actually works. That was definitively demonstrated in a ten-year project called the MacArthur Foundation Study of Aging in America, which was analyzed in John Wallis Rowe and Robert L. Kahn's 1998 book, *Successful Aging*. The study was a collection of dozens of individual research projects, all designed to "pinpoint the many factors that conspire to put one octogenarian on cross-country skis and another in a wheelchair." One study, for example, followed more than 1,000 high-functioning adults for eight years. Another project scrutinized hundreds of Swedish twins in an effort to determine how genetics and lifestyle played into aging. "There is a simple, basic fact about exercise and your health: fitness cuts your risk of dying. It doesn't get much more 'bottom line' than that," wrote two of the scientists who managed the project.

The study's authors debunked claims about DHEA, HGH, testosterone, and other anti-aging favorites, while laying out a litany of convincing evidence about the value of physical activity. Exercise cut the risk of developing coronary artery disease, diabetes, and colon cancer, they discovered. It slashed the chance of developing high blood pressure by half. And there was no need for seniors to engage in Mr. Universe–style bodybuilding or to spend hundreds of dollars consulting exercise physiologists. "Moderate physical activity, such as leisurely walking or gardening, was every bit as strong as strenuous exercise," they wrote.

Other studies proved that older people could enjoy the benefits of moderate exercise regardless of how late in life they started doing it. A study by the Institute for Aerobics Research in Dallas, Texas, followed 13,000 men and women for eight years. The researchers found that death rates dropped dramatically among people who stopped being couch potatoes and started taking half-hour walks a few times a week. The researchers also found that men who became fit decreased their risk of dying of any disease by 44 percent.

Many of the most famous examples of successful aging were people who shunned hormones and steroids. Fitness industry pioneer Jack LaLanne told Larry King in 2000, "I wouldn't take a steroid if you'd give me $10 trillion." He was 85 at the time and had chalked up an impressive list of achievements. In addition to founding a health-club empire (which he sold to Bally Total Fitness), he performed physical feats that most young people wouldn't dare to try. At 60 he swam from Alcatraz Island to Fisherman's Wharf in San Francisco, in handcuffs and shackles, towing a 1,000-pound boat. A decade later, handcuffed and shackled again, he towed 70 boats more than a mile from the Queensway Bridge in Long Beach, California, to the *Queen Mary.* He wanted everyone to know he didn't take any dangerous substances, not even prescription drugs. "You start fooling around with Mother Nature," he warned King, "you start taking all these supplements, all these artificial things— it's going to catch up."

But only a handful of anti-aging clinics actually offered exercise counseling. San Diego anti-aging doctor Ron Rothenberg was one of the few who prodded his patients to get fit. "Exercise is good for cognitive function, immune function," Rothenberg said in 2006. "Some people think they don't need it. I try to encourage it."

As part of a full-day anti-aging assessment, Rothenberg shuttled new patients to a gym a few miles away, where they were put through a battery of tests. Nutritionist and exercise specialist Robert Yang studied their posture and the strength of their abdominal muscles. He put blindfolds and noise-canceling earphones on them and then told them to march in place—a test designed to determine whether they were so far out of alignment that they'd actually walk right into a wall. Yang, an energetic Californian who shared a love of surfing with Rothenberg, told all his patients that everyone should lift weights to build a six-pack abdomen. He explained how they could do stretching exercises to properly align the spine, as he pointed to a poster on his wall labeled "The Human Spine Disorders."

Following the session with each new patient, Yang typed up a one-page evaluation and e-mailed it to Rothenberg. "Rounded shoulders, sway back posture," read one such evaluation. "Poor lower abdominal coordination, reduced range of motion of hip extensors." Rothenberg then gave patients lists of exercises that he believed they should do to correct their physical shortcomings. This part of his anti-aging plan was especially expensive: Rothenberg charged $400 for the one-hour fitness assessment with Yang, and another $300 for nutrition counseling. It was a lot to ask of patients, especially considering they could have purchased an hour with a personal trainer at the average gym for as little as $50.

"How are you feeling?" Rothenberg asked one patient who visited his office in 2006. "Good. I've been surfing," the patient replied, reporting that he had also been running and biking and that he got up every morning at 4:30 to do yoga. The 56-year-old teacher conceded that Rothenberg's program and exercise counseling had set him back a bit. "I have to put aside a certain amount of money for it, and sometimes I have to stretch things out to make ends meet," he said. "But I've noticed a difference. You get older, and your muscles get weaker. I don't know what I would feel like if I weren't doing this."

But most people seem hardwired to hate exercise. Even working out for a scant half hour is a lot to ask: A 2009 Gallup survey found that only one in four Americans were able to get off their butts for even that short a time, five or more days per week. And while anti-aging doctors claimed to care about how fit their patients were, most didn't place nearly as much emphasis on exercise as they did on hormones. "Well, we don't do any exercise here," said Houston anti-aging physician Steven Hotze. "The reason we don't is that on every corner in Houston you got a Bally's or you got a Gold's and every building's got exercise equipment in it. Most people when they come in say, 'My doctor told me to exercise. I don't have the energy to exercise.' Well, let's get your energy level up."

Given the choice between exercise and hormones, many patients took the easy way out. Just a few years after Yang started working with Rothenberg, he found that traffic from the San Diego anti-aging clinic had dried up.

Mainstream medical societies continued to warn patients away from the anti-aging industry and the hormones it promoted. At its 2009 annual meeting in June, the American Medical Association adopted a new policy on the use of hormones for anti-aging purposes. Based on reviews of dozens of scientific studies, the AMA's Council on Science and Public Health concluded in a report for the association's members: "Despite the widespread promotion of hormones as anti-aging agents by for-profit Web sites, anti-aging clinics, and compounding pharmacies, the scientific evidence to support these claims is lacking." It stated, "Current evidence fails to support the efficacy of HGH

as an anti-aging therapy and adverse events are significant."
Furthermore, the AMA's statement said, "No credible scientific
evidence exists on the value of so-called 'bio-identical hormones,' and there are concerns about their purity, potency and
quality because they are not approved by the FDA."

In December 2008, a few steps away from the rows of companies selling hormones and resveratrol and açaí supplements at
A4M's Las Vegas conference, BodyLogic's Patrick Savage dined
on oyster shooters and pricey red wine and marveled at how
far he had come since he and his brother founded their company five years earlier. Back then, he didn't have enough
money to stay in a room at the Venetian, where the conference
was held, so he shacked up in a cheap hotel on the strip. Now
he was a featured speaker, and his company was so profitable
he could afford to host a dinner for more than 25 of his doctors
and pharmacists at David Burke, one of the fanciest restaurants
in Vegas.

The country was going through the worst recession in 30
years, but BodyLogic wasn't suffering. "This is the perfect example of a service you're not going to give up in a bad economy," Savage said. "When you start working with a physician
to truly change your lifestyle, you make those hot flashes go
away, you can sleep again, your family actually likes you being
around, you're having fun, you're enjoying your libido. Patients make trade-offs. One gentleman gave up his F-150
pickup so his wife could be on hormones."

A few months later, Winfrey launched her series of specials
on longevity, and BodyLogic was officially "Oprah-whelmed,"
Savage said. As he dashed through his Boca Raton headquar-

ters, he remarked that he would have to abandon the office halfway into the lease, because BodyLogic no longer fit there. "We have 7,500 active patients now and we'll have 11,000 by the end of the year," he said. "Ever since Oprah hit, we're booking 4,000 patients a month. We moved here 14 months ago with seven employees." At 25 employees and growing, he said, he planned to move into a building twice as big. "My goal had always been 50 centers with 70 physicians. We're going to be well past that goal," he said breathlessly. "It's hard for me to even estimate now where we'll be in three years. It's hard to calculate the trajectory."

Then Savage showed a rare hint of self-doubt. "Do you think we act ethically?" he asked. But he didn't wait around for the answer. Instead, he went back to fielding calls from doctors who wanted to join BodyLogic and to building up the company's phone and computer networks, so it could handle the thousands of queries from prospective patients.

And despite the warnings, the customers just kept coming— eager to buy into the impossible dream that they, too, could take a swig from the fountain of youth.

ACKNOWLEDGMENTS

No one wants to hear that there's no such thing as a fountain of youth. That's why I'm so grateful to Basic Books, and especially my editor Tim Sullivan, for taking a chance and publishing a book that may be hard medicine for many people to swallow. Thanks also to Lorin Rees, for helping me develop the idea.

I could not have wrapped my brain around this topic without the help of many academicians, including John Hoberman, Sara Rosenthal, Tom Perls, and Larry Sasich. Thanks especially to Adriane Fugh-Berman and Jay Olshansky for walking me through the intricacies of hormone-replacement therapy and for reading the manuscript and helping me shape it.

I greatly appreciate the expertise of the many medical professionals who are not named in this book but who have been working tirelessly to educate the public about the risks of anti-aging medicine. Their insight was vital to completing this project.

Thank you to *Business Week* science editor Neil Gross, who recognized a good story and fought to get it on the cover.

And finally, thanks to all the doctors, pharmacists, scientists, and patients—on both sides of the anti-aging debate—who let me witness firsthand their fight against the inevitable passage of time and youth.

RESOURCES

It's easy to find books and Web sites extolling the supposed value of hormone-replacement therapy and other anti-aging remedies. It's harder to find the opposite view, however. Here are some sources that help compose a more complete picture of this field:

Butler, Robert N., M.D. *The Longevity Revolution: The Benefits and Challenges of Living a Long Life.* New York: PublicAffairs, 2008.

Columbia University Mailman School of Public Health. MacArthur Foundation Research Network on an Aging Society. http://aging societynetwork.org.

Growth Hormone/HGH/Anti-Aging and Sports. www.hghwatch.com.

Hoberman, John. *Testosterone Dreams.* Berkeley and Los Angeles: University of California Press, 2005.

International Longevity Center—USA. Publications: Healthy Aging. http://www.ilcusa.org/pages/publications/healthy-aging.php.

Mayo Clinic. Healthy Aging. http://www.mayoclinic.com/health/healthy-aging/MY00374.

———. Menopause. http://www.mayoclinic.com/health/menopause/DS00119.

National Research Center for Women and Families. http://www.center4research.org.

New England Journal of Medicine. Posting of Daniel Rudman study and accompanying warnings. http://content.nejm.org/cgi/content/short/323/1/1.

The Nurses' Health Study. http://www.channing.harvard.edu/nhs.

Olshansky, S. Jay, and Bruce A. Carnes. *The Quest for Immortality: Science at the Frontiers of Aging.* New York: W. W. Norton, 2001.

Olshansky, S. Jay, et al. "Position Statement on Human Aging." In "The Truth About Human Aging," *Scientific American*, May 13, 2002. http://www.scientificamerican.com/article.cfm?id=the -truth-about-human-agi.

Resveratrol: Separating Fact from Fiction. www.resforum.org.

Rowe, John Wallis, and Robert L. Kahn. *Successful Aging.* New York: Pantheon Books, 1998.

U.S. Food and Drug Administration (FDA). Pharmacy Compounding. http://www.fda.gov/Drugs/GuidanceComplianceRegulatory Information/PharmacyCompounding.

Women's Health Initiative. http://www.nhlbi.nih.gov/whi/.

INDEX